Heroin Century

D0208447

Heroin is a drug that myths are made of. Whether smuggled in the stomach of a camel or used as the ultimate symbol of lifestyle chic, no drug has been more argued over and legislated against, no drug has been more subject to misinformation and moral panic.

Heroin Century sets the record straight. It contains a wealth of historical and medical information about this drug which made its first appearance as a miracle medicine over a hundred years ago, and makes recommendations for its future in the twenty-first century. Evidence shows that heroin is dangerous principally because it is illegal. The authors argue that a more relaxed relationship between society and the drug would benefit both the economy and public health and safety.

Individual chapters describe the history of heroin production; the make-up of heroin and evolving methods of use; the spread of heroin and international efforts at control; typical 'career' patterns of users, ranging from occasional recreational use to destructive dependence; the subjective experience of taking heroin; the association between heroin and crime; the use of heroin in medicine and its effects on physical health; the history of the treatment of heroin dependence; and likely changes in heroin use in the future. The authors have drawn on literary and artistic sources as well as the large pool of scientific literature to compile a comprehensive and fascinating account of this world-changing drug.

Heroin Century makes available a wealth of information about the history, chemistry, pharmacology and medical aspects of heroin in a form accessible to anyone who wishes to participate in the contemporary debate about society's attitude to drugs.

Tom Carnwath is a Consultant Psychiatrist working with drug misuse services in Manchester. **Ian Smith** is an ex-heroin user, who has since trained in sociology and is now Service Development Manager for drug services in Manchester.

Heroin Century

Tom Carnwath and Ian Smith

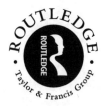

London and New York

First published 2002
by Routledge
11 New Fetter Lane, London EC4P 4EE

Simultaneously published in the USA and Canada
by Routledge
29 West 35th Street, New York, NY 10001

Reprinted 2002

Routledge is an imprint of the Taylor & Francis Group

© 2002 Routledge

The right of Routledge to be identified as the Author of this Work has
been asserted by him in accordance with the Copyright, Designs and
Patents Act 1988.

Typeset in Times by Taylor & Francis Books Ltd
Printed and bound in Great Britain by TJ International Ltd, Padstow,
Cornwall.

All rights reserved. No part of this book may be reprinted or
reproduced or utilised in any form or by any electronic, mechanical, or
other means, now known or hereafter invented, including
photocopying and recording, or in any information storage or retrieval
system, without permission in writing from the publishers.

British Library Cataloguing in Publication Data
A catalogue record for this book is available from the British Library

Library of Congress Cataloging in Publication Data
Carnwath, Tom
Heroin Century/Tom Carnwath and Ian Smith
p. cm.
Includes bibliographical references and index
1. Heroin. I. Smith, Ian, 1947 Apr. 7- II. Title.
HV5822. H4 C35 2002
362.29'3–dc21

ISBN 0–415–27871–6 (hbk) 0–415–27899–6 (pbk)

This book is dedicated to Ian's son Billy and to Tom's grand-daughter Artemis, in the hope that they will grow up in a world less polluted by drug racketeering. Also to Julia, heroine of Tom's half-century.

The sleep-flower sways in the wheat its head
Heavy with dreams, as that with bread:
The goodly grain and the sun-flushed sleeper
The reaper reaps, and Time the reaper.

From 'The Poppy' by Francis Thompson

Contents

Introduction and overview

Recently the following list of 'facts' about heroin appeared in a prominent position in a national newspaper.[1] Most of them were wrong.

Heroin: the facts

- Users agree that heroin is seductive, pernicious and now the most fashionable of all the so-called recreational drugs with the young. Diamorphine, to give the killer its clinical name, gives a sense of extraordinary well-being and security before relentlessly destroying every victim too weak to quit.
- Today the drug is easily available in every city and town in the country. And 'smack' is cheap too: at £20 a gram it is a third cheaper than its Class A rival, cocaine. The drug can be snorted, injected into veins or smoked – 'chasing the dragon'. Addiction is as inevitable as death and taxes.
- Main producers of the opium poppy, from which heroin is produced, include Turkey, Mexico, Iran and Lebanon. But the big fields are in the so-called Golden Triangle running from Laos through Cambodia and Burma.
- The hazards of heroin use are appalling: appetite loss, convulsions, vomiting, loss of bowel control, sleeplessness, rotting teeth, impotence in men, infertility in women and death.

Beside the list there was a photo of a long-haired man about to inject himself but already wearing the ecstatic expression of Bernini's *St Teresa*. The photo was clearly staged: the subject looked a bit like the young Mick Jagger and exuded 'heroin chic'. The syringe and needle, waved in the air as emblems, were clearly not intended for serious use. Rolled upwards, the eyes would definitely not have helped him inject successfully, particularly as he also handicapped himself by not wearing a tourniquet and by pointing his needle at ninety degrees to his arm rather than along the direction of the veins. The picture was more like an advertisement than a warning.

All this rather surprised us, because the paper in question often prints well-balanced articles on drug policy. But in truth we could have picked a hundred other examples of misinformation – from this paper and the rest of the press. We wrote to the editor pointing out that almost all the paper's 'facts' were just plain wrong, but he did not print the letter. We have therefore written this book instead.

Heroin is particularly good at inducing opinions which conflict with all the evidence and 'evidence' that is then moulded to fit the opinions. The drug problem appears so pressing, but the facts and the arguments are so contradictory and difficult. Even a brief dip in the swirling currents of the debate leaves one gasping for air and ready to cling to any opinion which might carry one to safety. Once aboard an opinion, people are understandably reluctant to jump off and start swimming again.

But even those who consider the evidence carefully can come to very different conclusions about the dangers of heroin and what action should be taken. We hope in this book to provide a dispassionate and objective review of heroin since its introduction to medicine about a century ago. Our main purpose is history and description, but inevitably our conclusions and beliefs will influence the flavour of the whole work. We will therefore state them in simplified form straightaway. Those who strongly disagree with us can stop reading at once and waste no further time. But we would like to point out, before they sign off, that we have come to these conclusions rather reluctantly and almost by surprise. We did not start out with these beliefs in any strong or coherent form but have slowly been persuaded by our research, experience and discussions.

Briefly, we believe that anxieties about heroin are exaggerated, that it is quite likely that it will be decriminalised or legalised in the not too distant future, and that when this happens it will not be a disaster. Health problems will perhaps increase, but not greatly. Street crime will probably decrease, but not greatly. There will, however, be huge economic benefits derived from cutting international gangsters out of the heroin market, abandoning this aspect of the 'war on drugs', and expanding legal trade and taxation revenue. We only discuss cannabis, cocaine and other illicit drugs in passing and do not offer any opinions about whether decriminalising these substances would be beneficial.

We are not writing an evangelical book and are not specifically concerned with persuading our readers. Our main aim is to provide accurate information. We believe that the debate about drugs should deal with each drug separately and should be based on knowledge about that particular drug. Each drug has different properties and history, and each has its own myths. Some are thought by many to be relatively harmless but are in fact dangerous, whereas others are thought to be very dangerous but in fact are not as bad as they seem. In our view ecstasy falls in the first category and heroin in the second.

We are constantly surprised how much of the debate on drugs is conducted on a platform of ignorance, even by those who are in charge of drug policy or are leading opinion-formers in the press or on television. We offer this book as a corrective and ask that there should be specific public discussion about heroin independently of other drugs. We predict that changes in attitudes to heroin will make a huge impact on our world in the next ten to twenty years and that therefore we need to start preparing ourselves now.

We are definitely not advocating the use of heroin. We believe it would be better if it had never been invented. We want to make absolutely clear our view that to start using heroin under present conditions would be immensely foolish. Dependence is easily acquired, and usually leads to huge grief both for users and their families. When we argue that heroin is potentially less dangerous than is often thought, we are referring to a possible future when pharmaceutical heroin can be acquired at a reasonable price, and safer methods have evolved for taking the drug. All this will be explained in later chapters. Current users of street heroin run risks which vastly outweigh any consolation provided by the drug. We are not advocating the legalisation of heroin at present. At a time when less than 1 per cent of the population has used the drug, it is premature to take such a step into the unknown. It is possible, but we believe unlikely, that heroin use will decrease, as it did in the United States in the 1930s and again in the early 1970s. In that case, most people will consider continued prohibition as justified. Our best guess is that use will continue to climb, and that in ten to fifteen years there will be a substantial constituency of heroin users, as large for example as the number of those who attend religious services regularly. At that time, most people will think that the costs of continued prohibition outweigh the benefits.

We come to heroin from quite different directions. Tom Carnwath has an establishment background, studying medicine at Cambridge and then in London. He worked as a GP briefly before training as a psychiatrist. He has the usual string of official-looking letters after his name. He did not think seriously about drugs at all until about twelve years ago, when a colleague resigned from his job, and then he found himself the only Consultant available to replace him, part-time, at the local drug dependence clinic.

In spite of years of training, you only seriously start learning in medicine when you begin to work in the specialty. He was lucky to find himself assigned to one of the best drug dependence teams in the country, both as regards skill and the friendly support of colleagues. Staff members patiently helped him find his feet and cover up his initial ignorance. Since then he has experienced an intensive but enjoyable education, delivered willingly by staff, patients and colleagues at other hospitals, and supplemented by feverish reading of the voluminous literature. He now works full-time as a Consultant in Addiction Psychiatry and has written many papers on opiate and stimulant addiction and related topics. He has no personal experience of heroin use.

While Tom Carnwath was tentatively dissecting a cadaver at the Cambridge Anatomy Department, Ian Smith was already deeply embroiled in the developing drug scene in both the North and South of England. An early 'drugstore cowboy', obtaining his supplies from pharmacy break-ins, he drifted into the London scene and eventually the tedium of life on a methadone prescription. Conflict with the law and the treatment system resulted in his break with opiates and the beginning of a long love affair with drink. He managed to give this up too for several years, but he has now finally mastered the art of moderate drinking. He remains defeated by nicotine, proving through a sample of one the oft-stated theory that cigarettes are harder to kick than heroin.

His experience of the treatment system led him back into working with drugs from the other side. After doing various voluntary jobs, he took a degree in sociology. He then helped organise a self-support group for drug users. Over recent years he has been working as a project officer in the same drug team as Tom. He has also been co-organiser of a diploma course in drug policy for local professionals and editor of a polemical magazine for drug users: *Monkey*. Both he and Tom share a similar age and a pleasure in debate, which has taken place in and out of work for at least five years. Out of this crucible have flowed the majority of ideas and thoughts expressed in this book.

We therefore look at heroin from different standpoints, one from inside and one from outside. One of us has trained in physiology and pharmacology, the other in sociology and criminology. One of us is by nature conservative and for the most part trustful of authority, the other radical and impatient of power structures. One is comfortably established, the other restless and usually on the move. The contrasts could be multiplied indefinitely. But both of us have a great deal of experience of heroin and its consumers. In spite of personal differences in attitude and philosophy, this experience has led over time towards a large measure of agreement in our debates on heroin. So much so that we now have to look for other topics to enjoy the cut and thrust of argument.

We find this comforting. It supports our view that our arguments are based not on our personal prejudices but on the history and properties of the drug. We think we can serve as triangulation points, allowing the observer to fix the position of heroin with confidence by noting its orientation to two widely separated landmarks. We feel confident at least that the fruits of this process are worth sharing with others. Most books on this subject are either strident and partisan, or densely academic. We hope that we have been able to write a book that is balanced, informative and easy to read.

We are writing specifically about heroin, which means that we are writing almost entirely about the twentieth century. We need to set the scene first, by describing very briefly the history of opiate use in preceding centuries. A number of good historians have tackled this subject, particularly the intriguing story of opium in Britain in the last century and the scandal of the Opium Wars.[2] We draw heavily on their work in the following account.

A brief history of opium

The principal active ingredient of opium is morphine. Heroin is a derivative of morphine, and in most pharmacological respects it is very similar. The main difference is that it is slightly more potent gram for gram, and it penetrates the nerve cells of the brain more rapidly. Opium has been with us almost forever, and up until about a century ago it had been consistently seen as one of the great benefits given to us by God. The Romans, for example, used it in a huge variety of tinctures, tablets, poultices and lozenges.

Modern use started with the famous sixteenth-century physician Paracelsus, who prescribed it to his patients mixed with alcohol and spices. He called this medicine 'laudanum' after the Latin word *laudandum*, something worthy of praise. Over the next 400 years it was a favourite medicine throughout Europe. In the eighteenth century, an English physician claimed that

> it causes promptitude, serenity, alacrity and expediteness in dispatching and managing business, assurance, ovation of the spirits, contempt of danger and magnanimity … it prevents and takes away grief, fear, anxieties, peevishness, fretfulness … it lulls, soothes and (as it were) charms the mind with satisfaction, acquiescence, contentation and equanimity.[3]

Clearly a very useful medicine!

It became particularly popular in Britain in the nineteenth century, where yearly opium consumption increased from one pound per thousand people at the beginning of the century to over ten pounds at the end. Until the Pharmacy Act of 1868 it could be sold or purchased by anybody. In 1850 twenty-five drops of laudanum could be purchased for a penny from the corner shop, the pub, the market stall or even from the enterprising lady next door. Opium was the aspirin of the day, and was the everyday treatment for every type of ill, be it headache, rheumatism or a touch of the nerves.

It had an important part to play in child-care. Mothers used it to keep their children quiet, particularly when they went out to work all day in the mills, but also at night so as not to aggravate their neighbours in the crowded tenements. One respectable Manchester pharmacist regularly supplied 700 households with a 'quietener' containing 100 drops of laudanum to the ounce, and was able to do nicely by selling five gallons a week. Other similar medicines rejoiced in names such as Mrs Winslow's Soothing Syrup and a Pennyworth of Peace. Laudanum was also good at treating diarrhoea, which was endemic in unsanitary living quarters and would have been life-threatening to young children. Apart from use in medicine and child-care, laudanum was a popular tipple, particularly in the Fens. Opium also formed a popular ingredient of sweet-cakes and lozenges enjoyed by children.

Friederich Serturner isolated morphine from opium in 1803 but it did not make a big impact in medicine for fifty years. All this changed with the invention of the hypodermic syringe in 1856. Morphine injections became a staple treatment in army field hospitals. The American Civil War turned a huge number of Americans into opiate addicts.

> Maimed and shattered survivors from a hundred battlefields, diseased and disabled soldiers released from hostile prisons, anguished and hopeless wives and mothers, made so by the slaughter of those who were dearest to them, have found many of them temporary relief from their suffering in opium.[4]

After the war, physicians found the morphine syringe an excellent way of treating patients already accustomed to opiates. Relief of pain was instantaneous. Of all the drugs in the doctor's bag, morphine became the most popular and was used for treating everything from nymphomania to vomiting in pregnancy. Concerns about widespread 'morphinomania', or morphine addiction, only surfaced at the end of the century. Opiate addiction has with some justice been dubbed the 'American Disease'.[5]

The Chinese did not have much tradition of opium use until about 1800. Doctors used it to a small extent in some areas of China as a painkiller and a remedy for dysentery. There was almost no history, however, of opiate addiction. Popular unfamiliarity with the drug was indicated by the Chinese word for opium, which translates literally as 'foreign medicine'. British traders were keen to purchase from China rice, silk, and above all, tea, which had suddenly become all the rage back in Britain, but they could find nothing which the Chinese wanted in exchange. When the East India Company took over Bengal in 1773, they also took control of some of the best opium fields in the world. Opium provided the answer to their trading problem. It was not long before opium started flooding into China. Since the Chinese had no familiarity with the drug, many soon developed serious addiction problems and the habit spread quickly inland.

Chinese emperors issued a number of decrees against opium but to no avail. In 1839 the Emperor's high commissioner confiscated a large quantity of opium and burnt it publicly in Canton. The international powers were affronted. The British sent a fleet and by 1842 the First Opium War was over. As a result of the Treaty of Nanking, China ceded Hong Kong to Britain, exclusive trade entry into five major ports and a large sum of money in compensation for British losses. The *Illustrated London News* boasted that the treaty 'secures us a few round millions of dollars and no end of very refreshing tea'.[6] In 1860 the Second Opium War forced China to legalise the use of opium altogether. Resentment against this humiliating episode contributed in time to the Boxer Rising, the rise of nationalism and the fall of the Manchu Dynasty.

By the end of the nineteenth century the Chinese authorities were able to take action against opium, principally because an active group had emerged in Britain which was campaigning against this abuse of imperial power. Doctors were also beginning to worry about morphine addiction at home. At the same time the Americans had become concerned about opium smoking, which Chinese workers had introduced on the West Coast railroads. They had also come face to face with opium in their new colonial role in the Philippines. We will explain later in the book how these and other influences led to various anti-drug conventions and treaties, and the start of an international drug control strategy.

As the twentieth century dawned, opiates were being consumed in large quantities in China and many other Asian countries, in most European countries and the United States. In other parts of the world they were used to a lesser extent. For most users they were a normal part of everyday life. We will describe how legislation reduced their use dramatically in Europe between about 1920 and 1975, but how they have made an unofficial comeback in the last quarter of the century. The United States suppressed opiates successfully for a period of about thirty years between 1920 and 1950, but much less successfully after that. The Chinese did not have much success until the Maoist revolution. Between about 1950 and 1980 there was probably little opiate use, although the figures are sparse and unreliable. Over the last twenty years it has been increasing steadily, in spite of draconian punishments. In most other Asian countries there was a gap of at most twenty years between the suppression of opium and its replacement by heroin.

We believe that the twentieth century has imposed only temporary interruptions on one of mankind's most ancient habits. Alfred McCoy, the distinguished historian of drug markets, predicts that within a generation world opium production will once again reach 40,000 tons, the amount produced at the beginning of the twentieth century before suppression got seriously under way.[7] Before many decades a pattern of use will probably establish itself again quite similar to earlier times. We will explain in the last chapter why we think this could happen rather quicker than most people expect.

Overview of contents

Heroin has been manufactured in many different ways since it first coalesced in a beaker at St Mary's Hospital, London, in 1874. In Chapter 1 we describe its journey downwards from the large pharmaceutical factories of Europe and Korea to the backstreet operators in Hong Kong and Mexico, and then on down to the saucepan and gas ring of the bedsit chemist. Enforcement activity has increasingly persuaded producers to prepare their heroin close to the poppy fields, in order to cut down on the costs and risks of transport. This causes huge environmental destruction, often in rich and fragile ecologies.

The way that heroin is produced and distributed means that users have no guarantee of the purity of what they purchase. The recent tragic deaths of about thirty British heroin users bear witness to this. A nasty bug called *clostridium novyii* had contaminated a consignment of imported heroin. It caused almost immediate sepsis on injection, with death one or two days later. All this caused minimal stir in the media compared to the huge coverage of the solitary death of Leah Betts from taking an ecstasy tablet.

Although it was not mentioned in the newspaper article's list of main producers, Afghanistan is by far the largest producer of heroin today. Places such as Turkey, Iran and Lebanon, which were once major producers, have not been so for many years.

In Chapter 2 we describe the different types of heroin, and the important difference between heroin prepared for smoking and for injection. The type of heroin found in Britain is not at all good for inhaling through the nose, or 'snorting', and so this practice is rare. On the other hand, it is a common method of use in the United States. The method of consuming heroin has changed radically over the course of the last century. In China eighty years ago the most popular method was to smoke little pink 'heroin pills'. 'Chasing the dragon' was only invented in Hong Kong in about 1950. It quickly proved popular, and spread rapidly through Europe, but has never made much headway in the United States except on the West Coast. Intravenous injection was first discovered by drug users in about 1925. Like most famous discoveries it appears to have emerged simultaneously in two separate places, Indiana in the US and Alexandria in Egypt. We describe why people choose to snort, inject or smoke, and how often they change between modes of consumption and the importance of this for health policy.

We describe the spread of heroin in Chapter 3, and efforts made by governments to resist its advance. Use and consumption were pretty much unregulated before World War I. British and European firms profited hugely from exporting tons and tons of heroin and morphine to addicts in the Far East. In between the wars, the League of Nations achieved some success in cutting back this industrial form of drug dealing. A frightening outbreak of heroin use in Egypt goaded them into making effective agreements, particularly the Statute of Limitations of 1935. But all this led to the establishment of illegal factories, which expanded rapidly after the end of World War II.

Since that time heroin production has been in the hands of gangsters and government action has had no success in reducing the supply. In general, purity has increased and the price has come down. In areas of common use in the UK, such as Liverpool, Manchester and Glasgow, the price has fallen over the last ten years from about £70 a gram to £45 a gram. It is much cheaper than it was but still nowhere near the newspaper's claim of £20 a gram. There is evidence that it is beginning to move upmarket and that there is growing interest among middle-class users looking for recreation. This is a very important trend, but it is absolutely not the case or even remotely the case that it is 'now the most fashionable of all the so-called recreational drugs with the young'.

One reason that heroin has spread is that governments have consistently treated national security as being more important than fighting drugs, whatever they might say in public. In our view this is quite reasonable in principle, although we might not see eye to eye with them on what constitutes national security in particular cases. The US Central Intelligence Agency formed a number of notorious alliances with major drug dealers in its war against communism. Nearly all the Western governments supported the Afghan guerrillas when they were fighting Russia. The most useful method of help was condoning their sales of heroin. The Taliban have been by far the largest suppliers of heroin in the world.[8] Over recent years gangsters have been increasingly aided by corrupt governments, and indeed in some countries they are the government. The extraordinary volume of illicit drug money already threatens the stability of the world's financial systems.

In Chapter 4 we consider the various patterns of heroin use and discuss whether it is useful to talk of a heroin 'career'. In spite of the claims of the article mentioned earlier, it is definitely not true that 'addiction is as inevitable as death and taxes'. The majority of people who use heroin do not become addicted, and indeed stop using it before they run that risk. Another substantial group continue to use it but take active steps to avoid physical dependence. Others become physically dependent, but because they are able to ensure a regular supply this is not a particular problem for them. Public perception of heroin use is overinfluenced by the image of a junkie, perhaps because this is the visible face of the habit. Controlled users are by nature discreet. It is only when the user gets into real trouble that he starts becoming a spectacle. Many users never descend into 'junkiehood'. Many others only do so as a short phase in a long career.

In Chapter 5 we look into the reasons why people use heroin. Works of writers such as William Burroughs, Alexander Trocchi and Ann Marlowe provide interesting insights. We consider why it has been so popular among musicians and whether or not it aids creativity. Investigators have recorded huge numbers of interviews with street users. Many users do not see it as a way of escape but something to help them get on with their daily life. It is, for example, a great drug to use when doing housework because it produces a sense of calm detachment and also quite often a feeling for order. The rituals of heroin preparation have much the same social significance as the more familiar ones associated with alcohol (buying a round, making a toast, drinks parties and so on). In this way heroin becomes a focus for fellowship.

In Chapter 6 we consider the relationship between heroin and crime. We argue that it has been exaggerated. It is certainly the case that heroin and crime are both prevalent features in the most deprived areas and so they often walk hand in hand. It is a small group of heroin users who commit most of the crimes and these people were mostly criminals before they started using heroin. A causal relationship is not proven, even though we argue that it is in the interests of many groups in society to think it is, including some of the addicts themselves.

We look at heroin as a medicine in Chapter 7, and also consider its effects on the body. Heroin is a very effective analgesic and it also has various other uses, including the treatment of heart attacks. Morphine is still a very popular medicine in hospitals throughout the world but, if morphine and heroin were compared objectively property by property, heroin would probably come out the winner. Doctors surrendered it reluctantly in the face of international pressure. In the US there was a strong movement twenty-five years ago to reintroduce it for terminal care, but this was defeated as a result of pressure from the drug agencies. Unfortunately the negative connotations of drugs of addiction and their accompanying bureaucratic regulations have together led to a terrible underuse of analgesia in the treatment of cancer and other painful conditions. In 120 countries, opiates are not used at all in pain control, even though there is no satisfactory alternative. It is now much easier to get hold of an opiate analgesic if you are hanging about the streets in Manchester than if you are dying of an agonising cancer in Africa. This is a scandalous side effect of international drug controls.

Heroin does not cause 'appetite loss, convulsions, vomiting, loss of bowel control, sleeplessness, rotting teeth, impotence in men, infertility in women and death'. It has no effect on the teeth, convulsions are rare and nausea only occurs occasionally in people not used to the drug. It certainly reduces the attractions of sex,[9] but there is no clear evidence that it cause impotence or infertility. So far from causing loss of bowel control, its most annoying effect is constipation.[10] We all die in the end but there is no evidence that heroin shortens the lifespan. In fact, it has almost no harmful effects on the body and can be taken over many years without risk to health.

However, heroin users do come to grief. They do so when they use infected injecting equipment or inject heroin of uncertain strength and purity. This is mostly a result of the drug being illegal. Many heroin users also die early because they take overdoses of heroin mixed with other sedative drugs, such as Valium and alcohol. We discuss how this happens and what can be done to stop it.

In Chapter 8 we look at treatments for heroin use, both gentle and severe. Every year a sizeable number of users give up their habit spontaneously, but unfortunately there is no clear evidence that treatment speeds up this process. For this reason many governments have encouraged the establishment of methadone clinics and needle-exchange programmes, with the rationale of keeping people safe with clean drugs and equipment until they are ready to move away from opiates. We consider the evidence and also the recent experiments with heroin prescription in Switzerland and Holland. Perhaps all this is a prelude to letting people buy their own supplies rather than having them purveyed by drug clinics. Treatment outcomes might change as more middle-class people take up the habit. There is considerable evidence that people from comfortable circumstances respond much better to treatment for alcohol and nicotine dependence, and there is no reason to think this would not be the case with heroin.

In Chapter 9 we look into the future. Heroin use has changed radically over the last century, and will undoubtedly change at least as much over the next. New methods of consumption might include aerosol inhalers, 'smart' needles, skin patches, ultrasound-operated implants and gas-powered syringes that blast powders painlessly through the skin. These smarter delivery systems may well speed the move upmarket that is already happening. New types of medical treatment will keep pace.

Attitudes to drugs are changing fast. In particular the line between licit and illicit drugs is becoming very blurred. Once these lines start to shift, they can move very quickly. Possession of small amounts of heroin for personal use is no longer illegal in Portugal, Spain and Italy. We explain why we think heroin may be decriminalised within the next ten years. We think that with or without legalisation there is bound to be a large increase in use, but this will not necessarily lead to a big increase in health problems. Full legalisation would produce immense benefits financially, for example by taking the trade away from gangsters and increasing revenue from taxation.

Acknowledgements

This book has emerged out of endless discussions with the inspirational staff at Trafford Substance Misuse Service in Manchester, where we both work. We would particularly like to thank the following, who have provided a wealth of knowledge, creative thinking and supportive fellowship: Mike Smith, Sarah Sparkes, Tim

Bottomley, Martin McGroarty, Jim Barnard, Karen Lee, Noel Craine and Chris Wibberley. Many other members of the team have been of great assistance, but there is not space to mention them all by name. A particular vote of thanks goes to John Brooke, our dedicated librarian, without whose sedulous quests for obscure literature this book would have been impossible. And of course we want to thank the people at the Service who have taught us the most: the many patients who have given us time to discuss with them their own experience of heroin use.

Notes

1   Thomas, Sean (1999) 'Just another upper class junkie', *The Times* (13 January): 17.
2   In this account we have drawn heavily on the following books and articles: Levinthal, C.F. (1985) 'Milk of Paradise/Milk of Hell – the history of ideas about opium', *Perspectives in Biology and Medicine* 28: 561–77; Hayter, Alethea (1988) *Opium and the Romantic Imagination*, Wellingborough: Crucible; Fay, P.W. (1975) *The Opium War 1840–1842*, Chapel Hill: University of North Carolina Press; Berridge, V. and Edwards, G. (1987) *Opium and the People: opiate use in nineteenth century England*, New Haven: Yale University Press; Terry, C.E. and Pellens, M. (1928) *The Opium Problem*, Montclair: Patterson Smith.
3   Jones, John (1700) *The Mysteries of Opium Revealed*, London: Richard Smith.
4   Day, Horace (1868) *The Opium Habit*, quoted in Terry and Pellens (1928).
5   Musto, D.F. (1999) *The American Disease: Origins of Narcotic Control*, New York: Oxford University Press, is an excellent history of American narcotic control.
6   Quoted in Fay (1975), p. 366.
7   McCoy, A.W. (2000) 'Coercion and its unintended consequences: a study of heroin trafficking in Southeast and Southwest Asia', *Crime, Law and Social Change* 33: 191–224.
8   Just as we were going to press, we heard of the terrible attack on the World Trade Centre in New York and of the projected allied campaign against the Taliban for harbouring Osama bin Laden. Unfortunately it was too late to alter our book, except to insert this footnote.
    It is unclear what effect the campaign will have on world supplies of heroin. Initially they will increase as the Taliban raises funds for fighting. Defeat of the Taliban may not affect the heroin trade greatly, because most of their rivals are equally implicated. But if Afghan production does decline, in the longer term this will at best lead to a temporary heroin drought before a corresponding increase in production in Burma and South America.
    What intelligence has shown is the vast extent to which terrorism is funded by the drug trade. This supports the opinions we express in Chapter 9. Terrorism is a much greater danger to humankind than drug misuse. The best way to undermine international terrorism would be to

deprive terrorists of their main source of revenue. One way to do this
would be through legalisation.

9 Ann Marlowe writes:

> Making love on dope was like changing a tire under water, I felt
> torpid and unmanoeuvrable, as if there was something I had to do
> but couldn't shake loose of in order to be there and come.

See Ann Marlowe (1999) *How to stop time. Heroin from A to Z*, London:
Virago Press, p. 265.

10 All opiates cause constipation. The old opium smokers used to talk about
a 'yen-shee baby'. 'Yen-shee' was the concentrated residue of opium that
formed inside the pipe bowl after smoking. A yen-shee baby was what was
produced with much travail after a long period of constipation. 'Wrap it
up in a towel and it'll live, it's a yen-shee baby.' See D.W. Maurer (1978)
'The argot of narcotic addicts', in D.W. Maurer and V.H. Vogel (eds)
Narcotics and Narcotic Addiction, Springfield: Chas. C. Thomas, pp.
273–327.

1   *Next add 5 ml human blood*
The manufacture of heroin

The invention of heroin

Bunsen's burner was not the only legacy of the great chemist. He could also be called the grandfather of heroin. It was his pupil Augustus Matthiessen who established the programme that led to its discovery. Both men had participated fully in the flowering of synthetic chemistry that took place in Germany, particularly in the second half of the nineteenth century. Throughout the century German scientists were unchallenged leaders in this field of science, starting with Serturner's original isolation of morphine from opium. Matthiessen brought this knowledge to England when he came to work as a lecturer at St Mary's Hospital, London. His chief English assistant was C.R. Alder Wright. Together they undertook a comprehensive exploration of codeine and morphine, synthesising hundreds of new compounds based on these molecules. Wright continued when Matthiessen retired. Their excitement still shines through the dry prose of the learned articles, as day by day they made substances that had never been previously created.

In early 1874, Wright was considering the effect of acetylation on codeine and morphine.[1] He added large amounts of acetic anhydride to morphine and applied heat. His description of what happened is as detached as you would expect in a scientific report.

> When morphine is brought into contact with excess acetic anhydride, tetra-acetylmorphine is produced, whether by heating a few hours at 100 degrees centigrade, or by leaving several days at room temperature. On adding sodium bicarbonate to the product dissolved in water, a precipitate is obtained, flocculent at first, but soon becoming crystalline.[2]

Looking over Wright's shoulder, the modern reader experiences a twinge of apprehension, as this portentous chemical clumps together and crystallises for the first time in history.

For we now know that this powder was not tetra-acetylmorphine at all.[3] At this date Wright was misinformed about the molecular structure of morphine, believing it to be a double molecule. Later analysis has shown that the new substance had two rather than four acetyl groups attached to each morphine molecule, and should therefore have been called diacetylmorphine.[4] This name was later abbreviated to diamorphine, and much later the substance was christened 'heroin'.

Wright did not concern himself overmuch with the use made of his new creations. For him, this was an exercise in chemical mapping, rather than practical medicine. After exhausting codeine and morphine, he moved on to the chemistry of Japanese camphor, and then to household soaps and fireworks. Nonetheless, some of his substances were tested on animals, in London and later in Edinburgh.[5] The investigators concluded that none of Wright's morphine compounds had any significant advantage over morphine itself. Diamorphine was therefore not used as a medicine in England until the German company Bayer marketed it as heroin in 1898.

The British frequently complain that they are good at making inventions, but bad at exploiting them. Other Wright creations included benzylmorphine, ethylmorphine and apomorphine. All had to wait many years before a medical use was found. None were used medically in Britain until reintroduced by German companies. When Bayer marketed heroin as a treatment for tuberculosis, it was other German firms that fought back by promoting benzylmorphine as Peronin and ethylmorphine as Dionin. Some Wright compounds had to wait longer. It was eighty years before the American writer William Burroughs proclaimed apomorphine to be the only effective cure for heroin addiction.[6]

Injured *amour propre* must have played a part in the lukewarm reception these medicines received in Britain, when they were trumpeted as German inventions in 1898. J.F. Macfarlan's, the Scottish pharmaceutical company, wrote in disgust to the *British Medical Journal*:

> The introduction and advertising of well-known esters of morphine under such fanciful names as 'peronin', 'dionin' & 'heroin' may mislead some members of the medical profession into the belief that they are new and proprietary preparations …. As a matter of fact, they are all prepared and supplied under their proper names by ourselves and other competent manufacturers.[7]

The complaint was not justified. Although Macfarlan's may have produced these substances as chemicals, there is no evidence that they sold them for medical use before the Germans stole their thunder.[8]

The Germans had in truth arrived at the formulation themselves. The end of the century was a creative time for medical chemistry. The German chemical industry had grown rich on aniline dyes. These had almost universally replaced natural dyes as colouring agents and could be made cheaply from the by-products of oil and gas manufacture. By 1890 this hegemony was under threat from increased competition and reduced access to primary materials. The companies wanted to diversify and find other outlets for their chemical production lines. Medicine was an obvious target. Many firms invested in state-of-the-art laboratories and competed to employ the top pharmaceutical chemists. In this flurry of activity, diamorphine was reinvented on at least two occasions.

Joseph von Mering became famous for discovering hypnotic barbiturates. In 1897 he was working for E. Merck of Darmstadt. He synthesised a number of opioid alkaloids including diamorphine. He was probably the first to test diamorphine on human subjects, but he was not particularly impressed. He thought that ethylmorphine was better suited for treating pain and tubercular coughs. Diamorphine was dropped and later that year Merck marketed ethylmorphine under the name of Dionin.[9]

Bayer was another large dye firm that had invested heavily in pharmaceutical research. Their laboratory was considered the most advanced in the world and they had had the good fortune to attract a chemist of growing reputation named Heinrich Dreser. Dreser was particularly interested in acetylation. He believed this process reduced the side effects of medications and also increased their potency. In 1894 Bayer had acetylated tannic acid which was used for the treatment of diarrhoea. They called the resulting compound Tannigen. It was less bitter than tannic acid and was also more effective. It quickly became popular among doctors and patients.

Encouraged by his success, Dreser set up a research group to investigate the acetylation of other medicines. The leaders in this group were Felix Hoffman and Arthur Eichengrun. In August 1897 they acetylated salicylic acid, producing the compound which was later called aspirin. Just a fortnight later they acetylated morphine and produced diamorphine, later called heroin. Within the space of two weeks they had created two new substances of astounding importance. Both could be leading contenders for the title of most important drug of the twentieth century.[10]

Of the two new compounds, heroin progressed most easily. Dreser was soon convinced of its power as a treatment for tuberculosis. He developed it quickly through animal and human testing, and brought it to the market in 1898.[11, 12] He thought it had a specific stimulatory effect on respiration, similar to that of digitalis on the heart, and he named it heroin in reference to the contemporary fashion for 'heroic' treatment, that is to say treatment that used powerful medicines in high doses.[13] He was clearly proud of his new medicine. He took the credit entirely for himself, failing to mention the work of Hoffman and Eichengrun or of earlier pioneers.

He was not convinced by aspirin and vetoed its further development. Had not Eichengrun ignored Dreser's instructions, aspirin might well have been abandoned and forgotten. It was only as a result of Eichengrun's unofficial action that its extraordinary properties were eventually recognised. It was finally also marketed alongside heroin in 1898. Even though Eichengrun played the more important part, Hoffman was credited by the firm with the invention of aspirin and for the most part still enjoys this reputation. The neglect of Eichengrun may have been a result of anti-Semitism. He was Jewish and later interned in Theresienstadt concentration camp.[14] Shortly before his death, he wrote a full account of his part in the discovery and development of aspirin. Understandably, he did not argue at this time that he was also the inventor of heroin. The subsequent history of the drug would have discouraged pride in this achievement. Nonetheless, Eichengrun has probably a good claim to the title, even if he did not want it.

Vats and funnels – industrial production of heroin

All the early makers of heroin basically used the same technique as Wright. They heated morphine with acetic anhydride and then used an alkali such as sodium bicarbonate to precipitate the powder. After its launch on the market, the manufacture of heroin was streamlined to enable industrial production but it still relied on morphine and acetic anhydride. Legitimate production increased rapidly, even after its use in medicine had become suspect. In spite of their initial scruples, British companies soon took over as the major producers. Companies such as Whiffens, T. & H. Smith and Macfarlan's made huge profits principally by exporting heroin and morphine to China, where it was mostly consumed by drug addicts. It was noted at the time that 'the Chinaman buys his morphia by the pound, and his predilection is for Macfarlan's, which he must have in original pound bottles'.[15]

It was certainly a scandal that European firms were capitalising so handsomely from Chinese drug addiction. To many it seemed that pharmaceutical trade was a continuation of the Opium Wars by other means. Pressure grew for action, spearheaded by the Americans who were concerned about their own problem of addiction and their newly acquired territories in the Philippines.[16] In 1912 the first international treaty was agreed and the first bricks laid in the increasingly cumbersome structure of international narcotic control.

As international controls started to bite, British production was reduced and Whiffens even had their manufacturing licence revoked following a smuggling scandal in 1923.[15] La Société Roessler et Compagnie, Mulhouse, took over for a time as chief producer. In 1928 it produced 4.35 metric tons of heroin, considered to be enough to satisfy the medical needs of the whole population of the world three times over. At the same time a Dutch company named Chemische Fabriek Naarden was actively importing and exporting heroin and cocaine through an underground network designed to evade the regulatory efforts of the League of Nations. The Opium Commission claimed that in 1928 it controlled over half the world production of heroin. The local authorities did not prosecute the company because they judged that although it had acted contrary to the spirit of the law, no single Dutch law had in fact been broken.[17]

Swiss companies have traditionally enjoyed more freedom from international conventions. Factories in Basle and Zurich plugged the gap as French production subsided. After the Swiss had bowed to international representations, production passed to a factory licensed to the French but operating in Constantinople. When this was closed by the Turks, the gauntlet was taken up by the Bulgarians. A new factory started up in Sofia. It is reckoned that this factory produced nine tons a year, mostly destined for the illicit market in Egypt and China.[18]

The Bulgarians in turn acceded to pressure, and suppressed this factory in 1931. Thereafter the Japanese became the major manufacturers and kept this dubious distinction right up until the end of the war. Heroin was distributed freely in the occupied Chinese province of Manchuria as an aspect of official policy. Not only did it produce a compliant population, but it also greatly enriched the Manchukuo Monopoly Bureau which was the only authorised supplier. Between 1934 and 1937, 94 per cent of world heroin production came from a Japanese factory in Seoul, Korea.[19] Japan at this time was aggressive and highly militarised. It was asserting its national identity after years of humiliation at the hands of Western powers. It was in no mood to bow to pressure from the League of Nations narcotic control programme. Indeed it had walked out of the League in 1931, after the League had condemned the Japanese invasion of Manchuria. It is ironic that in Japan itself heroin dependence was almost unknown.

It can be seen that there was little need for illicit production of heroin as long as the great trading countries of the world were taking turns to supply the burgeoning market created by heroin addiction. Nonetheless, some illicit production did begin in China before World War II, mostly in the region of Shanghai. After the war, the system of international controls passed to the newly formed United Nations in 1946. The Japanese were forced out of the market following their defeat in the war.

At long last, legitimate production of heroin was confined to supplying genuine medical need. World production plummeted and production was banned in many countries. Macfarlan's of Edinburgh had survived as heroin producers, having complied strictly with international treaties from about 1921. They took over once again as the world's leading licit manufacturer, a position which they have maintained until the present day. The amount they have produced since that time is tiny compared with their heyday around the time of World War I. It has been strictly for medical use in the few countries where heroin is still prescribed.

There was now a large number of heroin addicts, but no access to pharmaceutical heroin. Clandestine factories emerged across the world, for example in Turkey, France, Mexico, Greece, Hong Kong and the United States. By far the biggest producer at this time was the so-called Red Lion Company in Shanghai and its various offshoots. When the Communists took power in China, stringent penalties were imposed on drug trafficking. Most of the Shanghai chemists fled to Hong Kong and established their laboratories on British territory. This trade soon fell under the control of the Chiu Chau syndicate from Kwangtung, until their power base was weakened by huge drug seizures by the Hong Kong authorities in 1974. Many skilled heroin chemists left for Thailand and Malaysia from where they continued to export heroin into Hong Kong.[20] When enforcement became more effective in these countries during the 1980s, the chemists again moved on – to Myanmar, Laos, Pakistan and Afghanistan.

Today, the vast majority of heroin is produced in Afghanistan and the Golden Triangle, although there is also increasing production in Mexico and Latin America. In the East, a large number of the heroin technicians are direct descendants and apprentices of the original Shanghai chemists. Knowledge of their techniques will therefore give a good idea of how most of the world's illicit heroin is manufactured. Fortunately, both the Hong Kong Police and the US Department of Justice have provided detailed accounts based on their respective struggles with producers in Hong Kong and South-East Asia.[21] These give a graphic picture of the whole chain of production from the opium poppy through to heroin, along with details of all the reagents involved. The account is necessarily quite technical, but this is the only way to give some understanding of the struggle between producers and the authorities, and of the devastating damage to the environment that stems from unregulated production.

Oil drums and hammers – clandestine production

Opium production in South-East Asia is a family business. A typical family of poppy farmers ranges between five and ten people, including two to five adults. They will cultivate on average an acre of opium poppies per year. They usually plant cotton, tobacco and vegetables alongside the opium poppy for personal use. It is also common practice to plant maize and opium poppies in the same fields each year. The maize keeps down excessive weeds and provides feed for the farmer's pigs and ponies. It is grown from April to August. After harvesting the maize, and with the stalks still standing in the fields, the ground is weeded and prepared. Just before the end of the rainy season, in successive sowings throughout September and October, the poppy seed is sown among the maize stalks. The stalks protect the young opium poppy plants from heavy rains.

The opium poppy, *Papaver somniferum*, is an annual plant, ranging between two to five feet in height when mature. Under a microscope poppy seeds appear corrugated like peanut-shells. The seeds of the opium poppy can be distinguished by a fine fishnet pattern of ridges within the larger corrugations. The plant is hairless, unlike other poppies, and its leaves are arranged along the stem rather than at the base of the flowers. It grows best in temperate, warm climates with low humidity. It needs long days and short nights before it will develop flowers. Sandy loam soil suits it best, because such soil retains moisture and nutrients, is easily cultivated and supports healthy root development. Poppy plants can become waterlogged and die after a heavy rainfall in poorly drained soil. The best fields are therefore on mountain slopes 1,000 metres or more above sea level, with slope gradients of 20° to 40° to allow easy drainage of rainwater. Good fields can support opium poppy cultivation for ten years or more without fertilisers, irrigation or insecticides, before the soil is depleted and new fields must be cleared.

The poppy generally flowers after about ninety days of growth and continues to flower for two to three weeks. The petals last for two to four days and then drop to reveal a small, round, green fruit, which continues to grow. Only this pod portion of the plant can produce opium alkaloids. The skin of the poppy pod encloses the wall of the pod ovary. The plant's latex (opium) is produced within the ovary wall and drains into its middle layer through a system of vessels and tubes. The cells of the middle layer secrete more than 95 per cent of the opium when the pod is scored and harvested.

Most opium poppy varieties produce three to five mature pods per plant. A typical opium poppy field has 60,000 to 120,000 poppy plants per hectare, with a range of 120,000 to 275,000 opium-producing pods. The actual opium yield will depend largely on farming skill and weather conditions. The farmer and his family generally move into the field for the harvest, setting up a small hut on the edge of the poppy field. The scoring of the pods (also called 'lancing', 'incising' or 'tapping') begins about two weeks after the flower petals fall from the pods. A set of three or four small blades of iron, glass or glass splinters bound tightly together on a wooden handle is used to score two or three sides of the pod in a vertical direction. If the blades cut too deep into the wall of the pod, the opium will flow too quickly and will drip to the ground. If the incisions are too shallow, the flow will be too slow and the opium will harden in the pods. A depth of about one millimetre is ideal for the incision. Early the next morning, the opium gum is scraped from the surface of the pods with a short-handled, flat, iron blade seven to ten centimetres wide. Opium harvesters work their way backwards across the field scoring the lower, mature pods before the taller pods, in order to avoid brushing against the sticky pods. The pods continue to produce opium for several days. Farmers will return to these plants – sometimes up to five or six times – to gather additional opium until the pod is totally depleted. The opium is collected in a container, which hangs from the farmer's neck or waist.

The opium yield from a single pod varies greatly, ranging from 10 to 100 milligrams of opium per pod. The average yield per pod is about 80 milligrams. A typical opium poppy farmer household in South-East Asia will collect three to nine kilograms of opium from a year's harvest of a one-acre field. The opium will be dried, wrapped and stacked on a shelf by February or March. If the opium has been properly dried, it can be stored indefinitely. Part will then be kept for family use and the rest sold on to local morphine laboratories.

Opium sold to the laboratory undergoes more complex processing. It is mixed up with water and lime is added. This makes the coarse vegetable matter sink to the bottom of the tank, where it can be easily filtered away. Ammonium chloride is then added, which causes crude morphine to emerge from the solution. Crude morphine is a brown granular powder, which usually contains about 85 per cent morphine and 15 per cent codeine. It could be mistaken for coffee, if it wasn't for the distinctive smell of opium.

Hydrochloric acid is added to this powder to form morphine chloride. After further purification with powdered charcoal, the morphine chloride is ready for pressing. The wet powder was traditionally pressed in moulds to form rectangular blocks weighing just over a kilogram. Each processing plant had its own moulds decorated with distinctive trademarks: '999' was a common mark, which merely indicated that the product was morphine. This was usually combined with other symbols, which revealed to the initiated the place of origin.

The morphine blocks were traditionally sent on to Shanghai or Hong Kong for further processing. They became the main ingredients for the specialist heroin cooks[22] in their makeshift street laboratories. Their first job was to break up the blocks by a mixture of hammering and grating. They then slowly heated the morphine chips to remove all moisture and afterwards mixed it with acetic anhydride in large steel drums. This was an industrial-scale version of the original process used by Alder Wright at St Mary's. Unfortunately the ensuing reaction released quantities of pungent gas. Cooks had to use tight-fitting lids sealed with damp towels to avoid detection by police or neighbourhood informers.

When the reaction died down, water was added to convert any remaining acetic anhydride to acetic acid. Impurities were removed with chloroform. Next came the process of titration. Sodium carbonate was added to ensure neutralisation of the acetic acid. While this happened, the mixture tended to foam up and boil over, so it had to be carried out very slowly. All this time, the pH of the liquid was being measured with litmus paper, until the acid was completely neutralised.

The precipitated powder was filtered and dried. Mixers such as quinine, strychnine and scopolamine were added to give a characteristic flavour and feel. If heroin hydrochloride rather than heroin base was required, it was now necessary to add hydrochloric acid. To achieve a pure product was a complex process. Highly skilled cooks were responsible for preparing the famous Chinese No. 4 , which was almost pure heroin hydrochloride.

They first passed impure heroin hydrochloride over and over again through activated charcoal filters until it became colourless. They then added concentrated hydrochloric acid. Very slowly they poured in ether and propyl alcohol, stirring all the time with a bamboo spoon. They knew the right amount of ether had been added because the mixture would start to flash 'like shooting stars'. A white powder would settle to the bottom of the tank. They laid it out on trays and dried it with lime before distributing it for sale.

The manufacturing process sounds simple, but in fact it is difficult and dangerous. Heroin cooks are not skilled chemists, but usually apprentices that have learnt their trade by watching their teachers. They follow recipes that look more suitable for a kitchen than a scientific laboratory. The recipes are jealously guarded and either passed down through families or sold at a high price. Cooks are reluctant to change successful recipes, which probably accounts for the persistence of flavouring agents such as quinine and strychnine. The speed of heating, the temperatures achieved at different times, the waiting times left between the separate operations – these are all critical to successful manufacture. When effective police action causes expert cooks to leave an area of production, a rapid deterioration in heroin quality often follows as amateur cooks try to fill the gap. This happened in Hong Kong in 1974 and more recently in Mexico.

Reagents and precursors

Most of the chemicals involved pose particular risks. Acetic anhydride is a pungent colourless liquid that brings tears to the eyes. It may be difficult to obtain. If it is replaced with other reagents, such as acetyl chloride or acetyl bromide, there is a risk of explosion. Ether is highly inflammable. If it is brought too near the fire or overheated, the cook may disappear along with his laboratory. This is most likely to occur if cooks try to recover ether after heroin manufacture by distilling it out of the residual fluids. Hydrochloric acid is corrosive and can cause serious burns if it comes in contact with the skin. Hot liquid burns are also common, as the mixture boils up when the sodium carbonate is added. Cooks work with little or no ventilation in order to prevent the characteristic odours reaching the street. They often suffer eye and lung damage from the toxic vapours. It is not surprising that in a number of cases the police have only discovered a particular laboratory when it has exploded.

Apart from the morphine, most of the necessary ingredients are freely available. The exception is acetic anhydride, which falls under regulation through an international convention on 'precursors'.[23] Whereas coca and opium are nearly always grown in underdeveloped areas, precursors are usually manufactured by advanced industrial nations.

The International Narcotics Control Board (INCB) manages a programme for regulating the distribution of potential drug precursors, based on a convention from 1988. Precursor control is an important strand in their strategy because it is much easier to police precursor production and distribution in Europe and America than it is to control opium production in Afghanistan, Myanmar and Mexico.

A recent success for this programme has been Operation Purple, which was designed to control the production and sale of potassium permanganate. This dark purple powder leads a twilight life as an important component in the manufacture of cocaine. During a period of six months in 2000, almost 1,200 tons of suspicious shipments of potassium permanganate were intercepted, often travelling from Europe to South America.[24]

The INCB admits that the control of acetic anhydride has been much less satisfactory. They are aiming to mount an intensified operation against this precursor and to upgrade its scheduling under the 1988 Convention on Precursors.[25] There are a number of problems with this plan. Drug makers are not entirely dependent on industrial suppliers. Home chemists can produce acetic anhydride, although the process requires a certain amount of care and skill.[26]

The process is quite sophisticated, but well within the range of modern drug barons, particularly when they have government backing or are part of the government themselves. In the Central Asian republics that used to belong to the Soviet Union, whole chemical factories have been turned over to the production of acetic anhydride and other precursors. Thirty-eight countries have still not signed the 1988 Convention (fourteen in Africa, eight in Asia, six in Europe and ten in Oceania).

The INCB in its latest report requests them all to come aboard, somewhat in the tone of a tired schoolteacher:

> We reiterate our request to those States that have not already done so to take, as a matter of priority, the necessary steps to put into effect the measures required under the 1988 Convention and to accede to it as soon as possible.[23]

The tone of the request is polite, but it is backed up with heavy diplomatic pressure. Nonetheless, in a turbulent world, total compliance is a pipe-dream. Heroin manufacturers are no longer dependent on a supply of precursors from developed countries that comply with international treaties. As is often the way with embargoes, the major effect of the Convention on Precursors has been to increase self-sufficiency at ground level.

Drugs and the environment

Another effect of narcotic control has been to drive the total process of manufacture closer to the sites of opium cultivation. Processed heroin is easier to transport than morphine blocks. Profits are higher if cultivating regions can sell heroin rather than morphine. In this way opium cultivation itself is pushed towards remote areas where the ecosystem is often fragile. George Giacomelli, head of the International Drug Control Programme, graphically pointed out the drastic effects of all this on local ecology at the United Nations Environment Conference in Rio de Janeiro:

> Recourse to drugs is both the expression and the cause of a disruption of the ecosystem. Clandestine cannabis, coca and poppy growers penetrate into more and more remote and more and more fragile forest environments. These growers are often migrants from the most impoverished slums of megacities. They have no real agricultural experience, and unlike traditional farmers, they have no respect for the earth, which surrounds and supports them. Forests are destroyed manually, mechanically or by fire. No vegetation survives to stabilise or renew the soil. Land is used until its complete exhaustion. There is rapid erosion of soil. Fertilisers, pesticides, herbicides have a disastrous impact on tropical ecosystems. The operators of clandestine heroin and cocaine laboratories dump thousands of tonnes a year of highly toxic chemicals into water courses. Many rivers have already lost all trace of flora and fauna ... . Poppy cultivation has destroyed the ecological equilibrium of the Golden Triangle. Similar destruction has been wrought in the Golden Crescent in North Pakistan and Afghanistan. Uncontrolled deforestation has worn out the soil. Heroin trafficking now occurs also in the Chiapas tropical forest of Mexico, San Marcos in Guatemala, in many departments of Colombia and in the Maranon region of Peru.[27]   ·

These are all regions with a rich but fragile ecology. Already they have suffered significant depletion of biodiversity. Forests are cut down to enable opium growth, but the opium poppy rapidly exhausts the thin forest soils. Often they only sustain two to three crops before the site is abandoned and more forest is destroyed. In Laos it is calculated that 250,000 to 350,000 hectares of forest are lost to opium production every year.

In Latin America, opium poppies are usually planted in well-watered, steep-sloped mountain canyons or in small isolated stream valleys to limit visibility and prevent detection. These fragile habitats have been severely contaminated by chemicals such as lime, ammonia, tartaric acid, ammonium chloride, alcohol, acetone, acetic anhydride and hydrochloric acid. Fast-flowing rivers spread the pollution, which now threatens regional water resources.[28] About 6,000 tons of opium are produced in the world each year. Because heroin manufacture is for the most part illegal, it is totally uncontrolled. Traditional opium producers have received incentives and international aid to change their crops, with some limited success in civilised regions. Their place is filled by cowboy producers who are laying waste the most beautiful regions of the world for the sake of temporary profit.

Bathtubs and gas-rings – domestic production

Against this gloomy background, some acknowledgment must be made of the small-time cottage industries that have supplied morphine and heroin in regions cut off from international trade. Through much of the period of Soviet occupation, a dedicated band of addicts in Poland obtained their supplies by processing poppy straw. Ever since morphine was isolated, it has been known that poppy stalks contained morphine in small concentrations, but it proved quite impractical to extract it. It took a hundred years of experimentation before Jan Kabay discovered an economic method and established his morphine production company Alkaloida in the market town of Tiszavasvari in Hungary. The statue of Kabay inspecting his test tube still dominates the town square.

At first the technique involved processing the fresh stalks shortly after the poppies had flowered. By 1931 he had discovered how to process ripe dry stalks using extracting machines at the harvesting sites.[29] When this technique was developed, it caused great anxiety among those responsible for narcotic control. They feared it would lead to an increase in addiction. Poppy straw is easily obtained in poppy-growing regions. Perhaps addicts would be able to extract their own morphine using Kabay's method, and control would be impossible. After consideration, this anxiety was discounted. It was thought the process was so complicated it could only be carried out in sophisticated factories.[30]

The Poles proved the experts wrong. In 1976 an anonymous pharmacology student from Gdansk devised a method of extracting morphine from poppy straw using saucepans, bathtubs, gas-rings and other normal domestic equipment. This was called 'Polish heroin', even though at first it only contained morphine and codeine. The method soon spread to other Eastern bloc countries. It was named *chornyi* in Ukraine and *chimiya* or *hanka* in Russia. Poppy straw was also smuggled into Austria to make the locally valued 'poppy-head soup'. Up until the last decade, opiate use was rare in Poland. Most users belonged to small-scale cooperatives that manufactured their own heroin. Drug-related crime and drug trafficking for profit were practically unknown.[31]

All this changed after the fall of the Iron Curtain and the advent of a 'free market' economy. In the countries which once belonged to the Eastern bloc, injecting drug use became much more common and along with it came the epidemic spread of HIV infection. Acetylation of poppy straw morphine became popular, using the most basic bathtub technology. A bizarre feature of many drug kitchens is the use of human blood as an ingredient. The rational explanation is that chemicals are expensive and human blood acts as an effective neutralising agent. Five millilitres of fresh blood are apparently needed to neutralise a glass of poppy straw liquid. The practice may also owe its origin to a subconscious belief that human blood enhances the potency of injected drugs. Either way, a 'drug boiler' who wanted to start an HIV epidemic could not do much better than enrich his *hanka* with his own infected blood.[32]

Poppy-head infusions were used in Britain in the nineteenth century. The habit continued among a few enthusiasts until recently. Through a loophole in the drug laws, it was still legal to sell poppy heads in pharmacies right up until 1978. In 1981 a chemist was prosecuted for selling 300 poppy heads at a time to a single customer. He had prudently stocked up with 30,000 poppy heads shortly before the new regulations were passed.[33] Occasionally people still approach health services suffering from poppy-tea dependence.[34] There is no record, however, of heroin being prepared domestically from poppy heads or poppy straw in Britain.

There is however a suspicion that illegal heroin manufacture is starting to occur in Britain, using imported ingredients. Britain is the hub of European drug distribution. No secret refineries have yet been discovered, but on at least two occasions customs officers have intercepted shipments of acetic anhydride destined for the UK. A cargo of five tons was seized in Sri Lanka and one of three tons in Kenya.[35] It is a fair assumption that Customs intercept about 10 per cent of what gets through. If this is the case here, some eighty tons of acetic anhydride have already arrived in the UK, enough to make an awful lot of heroin.

Another example of isolation stimulating ingenuity comes from New Zealand. For many decades there was almost no access in these islands to international sources of heroin. Amateur chemists developed an advanced skill in converting over-the-counter codeine into morphine and then into heroin. This is named 'homebake'.[36] Similar techniques have been found in clandestine laboratories in Australia.[37] Homebake remains an important source of supply for New Zealand addicts. A few have also became adept at cultivating and harvesting opium poppies.[38] This type of pioneering self-sufficiency is rather reassuring when compared with the global heroin market and its unbridled drive towards crime, corruption and exploitation. It is only recently that foreign heroin has begun to make an impact on the New Zealand market.

Some traditional healers have also discovered fortuitously that acetylating morphine increases the efficacy of their remedies. The Hmong people of South-East Asia are traditional cultivators of opium and also practise a sophisticated form of folk medicine. Hmong refugees in the United States have been found in possession of 'backache medicines' which resemble charcoal in appearance. Analysis revealed a complex mixture of aspirin, paracetamol, caffeine, opium and heroin. (The first three ingredients are found in Britain in over-the-counter painkillers such as Anadin Extra.) Folk doctors apparently dissolve this kind of tablet together with opium and heat the mixture over several hours. In the process some acetylation of morphine takes place, so that the medicine ends up containing significant amounts of heroin. Patients were neither aware that the medicines contained heroin, nor that they were infringing US laws.[39]

Back to the vat – heroin production in the future

Narcotics control has enjoyed undoubted successes. The downside has been that drug production has been driven step by step away from organisations that can be policed and audited towards those that are inept and unprincipled. International control usually aims to increase the quality and reliability of manufactured products. In the case of heroin, it has had exactly the opposite effect. Up until World War II, nearly all heroin manufacture took place in approved pharmaceutical factories. Nowadays it nearly all takes place in unregulated workshops, set up for instant profit by ruthless gangsters. Volume of production has increased, industrial pollution has increased and quality has deteriorated. This chapter has chronicled the gradual transfer of production from the vats and beakers of the chemical laboratory to the oil drums of the clandestine chemist and the saucepans and bathtubs of the home producer. Fortunately, there have recently been some small signs of movement in the opposite direction.

Over the last few years, there has been some slight increase in the production of pharmaceutical heroin. For many years, it was almost entirely produced by Macfarlan's of Edinburgh, principally for use in Britain, both as a painkiller and as a treatment for a small number of heroin addicts. Recently there have been trials of heroin prescription for addicts in other countries such as Switzerland and Holland. Trials have also been contemplated in Canada, Australia, Germany and Spain. Heroin is being manufactured again in Belgium. The outcome is still uncertain, but it may indicate a trend towards eventually providing heroin users with safe and proper medication. This will be good for users, good for the environment and bad for the drug barons.

Notes

1   Acetylation is a key process in the manufacture of heroin, so a technical explanation is necessary here. It means altering a molecule by adding the 'acetyl' configuration of carbon, hydrogen and oxygen. The acetyl group is also denoted by the chemical formula CH_3CO. It is the first of a series of similar groups, including 'ethyl' (C_2H_5CO) and 'propyl' (C_3H_7CO). Under the right circumstances ethyl may break down to acetyl compounds, as happens when old wine turns into vinegar.

2   Wright, C.R.A. (1874) 'On the action of organic acids and their anhydrides on the natural alkaloids', *Journal of Chemical Society* 12: 1,031–43.

3   'Tetra' means 'four', so tetra-acetyl means four acetyl groups.

4   Lerner, M. and Mills, A. (1963) 'Some modern aspects of heroin analysis', *Bulletin on Narcotics* 15: 37–42.

5   Stockman, R. and Dott, D.B. (1890) 'Report on the pharmacology of morphine and its derivatives', *British Medical Journal* 5: 189–92.

6   Burroughs was champion and frequent partaker of the apomorphine cure for heroin addiction invented by the British physician Dr John Yerbury Dent, but which has since disappeared. See J.Y. Dent (1952) 'Apomorphine in the treatment of addiction to "other drugs"', *British Journal of Addiction* 50: 43–5. Although Burroughs achieved periods of abstinence after these treatments, he finally gave up heroin at the age of 66, when he went on a methadone programme. He described this as like switching 'from whiskey to port wine'. He was still in good health at that time. See Ted Morgan (1991) *Literary Outlaw*, London: Bodley Head, pp. 562–3. Rolling Stone Keith Richards kicked his heroin habit after undergoing apomorphine treatment.

7 Messrs J.F. Macfarlan & Co. (1899) 'Heroin etc.' (letter), *British Medical Journal* 1 (18 March): 675.
8 We are very grateful to Dr Harry Payne of Macfarlan Smith for consulting the firm's archives for us. He could find no evidence of the sale of diamorphine before 1898. However, he writes:

   It is quite probable that the product was sold. Unfortunately none of the price lists for this period have survived to support the idea. (One could possibly refer to Pharmacy Journals of the time to see if they advertise the product.)

   We have consulted the relevant pharmacy journals, but have found no mention of the sale of diamorphine in this period.
9 Mering, J. von (1898) 'Physiological and therapeutic investigations of some morphine derivatives', *The Merck Report* 7: 5–13.
10 Sneader, W. (1998) 'The discovery of heroin', *Lancet* 352: 1,697–9.
11 Dreser, H. (1898) 'Ueber die wirkung einiger Derivate des Morphins auf die Athmung' ('On the effect of some morphine derivatives on respiration'), *Archiv für Physiologie* 72: 485–521.
12 Dreser, H. and Floret, T. (1898) 'Pharmakoligisches ueber einige morphinderivative' ('Pharmacology of some morphine derivatives'), *Therapeutische Monatschefte* 12: 509–12.
13 Ridder, M. de (1994) 'Heroin: new facts about an old myth', *Journal of Psychoactive Drugs* 26: 65–8.
14 Sneader, W. (1997) 'The discovery of aspirin', *Pharmaceutical Journal* 259: 614–7. Initially heroin could be obtained over the counter, whereas aspirin required a doctor's prescription.
15 Parssinen, T. (1983) *Secret Passions, Secret Remedies*, Manchester: Manchester University Press.
16 See Chapter 3.
17 De Kort, M. and Korf, D.J. (1992) 'The development of drug trade and drug control in the Netherlands: a historical perspective', *Crime, Law and Social Change* 17: 123–44.
18 El Hadka, A. (1965) 'Forty years of the campaign against narcotic drugs in UAR', *Bulletin on Narcotics* 17: 1–13.
19 'History of heroin', *Bulletin on Narcotics* 5 (1953): 3–16.
20 Confidential report of the Royal Hong Kong Police Narcotics Bureau (1973) *Heroin Manufacture in Hong Kong* (September).
21 Confidential report of the Royal Hong Kong Police Narcotics Bureau (1973) *Heroin Manufacture in Hong Kong* (September); Drug Enforcement Administration (Intelligence Division) (1993) *Opium Cultivation and Heroin Processing in Mainland Southeast Asia*, Washington, D.C.: US Dept of Justice, Strategic Intelligence Section.
22 'Cook' is a better term than 'chemist', for most of these experts were quite unqualified and had no understanding of chemical reactions.
23 A precursor is a chemical that is required for producing an illicit drug.
24 International Narcotics Control Board (2000) *Report for 1999*, Vienna: United Nations.
25 United Nations (1988) *United Nations Convention Against Illicit Traffic in Narcotic Drugs and Psychotropic Substances*, Vienna: United Nations.

26 Vaporised acetone is passed across a heated filament to produce ketene, which is then allowed to react with glacial acetic acid. Alternatively, a ferocious reaction can be generated by dripping phosphorus trichloride into sodium acetate. Constant shaking and cooling is necessary. The reaction produces acetic anhydride, which is then purified by fractional distillation.

27 Giacomelli, G. (1992) 'UN executive statement at UN conference on the environment and development, Rio de Janeiro, 4/6/92', *Bulletin on Narcotics* 44: 3–7.

28 Armstead, L. (1992) 'Illicit narcotics cultivation and processing: the ignored environmental drama', *Bulletin on Narcotics* 44: 9–20.

29 The machines contained sodium bisulphite, which was used to concentrate the morphine through an elaborate 'counter-current' flow system. The resulting fluid was treated with alcohol and then the morphine was precipitated using ammonium sulphate in the presence of benzene. It was then purified by repeated recrystallisation.

30 Bayer, I. (1969) 'Manufacture of alkaloids from the poppy plant in Hungary', *Bulletin on Narcotics* 12: 21–9.

31 Watson, P. (1991) 'Supply and demand: lessons from Poland', *Druglink* (July–August): 12–13.

32 Rhodes, T. *et al.* (1999) 'HIV infection associated with drug injecting in the newly independent states, East Europe: the social and economic context of epidemics', *Addiction* 94: 1,323–36.

33 Anderson, S. and Berridge, V. (2000) 'Opium in 20th century Britain: pharmacists, regulation and the people', *Addiction* 95: 23–36.

34 Unnithan, S. and Strang, J. (1993) 'Poppy tea dependence', *British Journal of Psychiatry* 163: 813–14.

35 Observatoire Geopolitique des Drogues (1999) *Annual Report 1997–1998*, Paris: OGD.

36 The most frequently used chemical procedure is to demethylate the codeine by heating strongly with pyridine and concentrated hydrochloric acid. The resulting reddish-brown mixture is made alkaline with sodium hydroxide and the morphine is then extracted with chloroform. See K. Bedford (1987) 'Illicit Preparation of Morphine from Codeine in New Zealand', *Forensic Science International* 34: 197–204.

37 *Health Series Number 21: Illicit Drug Samples Seized in the Australian Capital Territory 1980 to 1997* (1998) Canberra: Australian Institute of Health and Welfare.

38 Hannifin, J. (1997) 'Where to next?', *Addiction* 92: 687–8.

39 Smith, R.M. and Nelsen, L.A. (1991) 'Hmong folk remedies: limited acetylation of opium by aspirin and acetaminophen', *Journal of Forensic Sciences* 36: 280–7. Acetaminophen is another name for paracetamol.

2 From mouth-organs to bazookas
Varieties of heroin and their use

There are as many varieties of heroin as there are types of tea. As with tea, consumers in one area are often unaware that different varieties and ways of use are commonplace elsewhere in the world. In Britain, until recently, tea users considered tea to be an infusion in boiled water of cheap dried tea-bush leaves, to which cold milk and usually sugar were added. Most were unaware of specific brands, such as Lapsang Souchong or Orange Pekoe; or green tea or brick tea; or tea boiled up with sweetened milk or with mint; or tea used in cooking to make ice cream or to flavour stews. They had no idea that these uses of tea were routine in other cultures.

With the advent of supermarkets and global marketing, 'tea consciousness' has increased. Most people have become aware of different varieties of tea. This is not the case with heroin. Heroin remains in a pre-supermarket state. Users only know about preparations sold in their home district. Different brands are not advertised or marketed on the Internet. This could well change in the near future, but at the moment methods and types of heroin use remain localised. Most users do not know the extent to which heroin has varied over time and place. This variety has been all the greater because, unlike tea, heroin is not only taken by mouth. It can also be sniffed, smoked and injected, and each way of use is best served by its own brand of drug.

Soothing mixtures

Most types of heroin are formulated with either heroin base or heroin hydrochloride. Heroin base is pure diamorphine. Heroin hydrochloride is what is called a 'salt' of heroin, produced by reacting it with hydrochloric acid. Initially there was only one preparation of heroin, namely pure diamorphine base, described in the *Lancet* as a 'white crystalline powder soluble in spirit but insoluble in water'.[1] It was bitter in taste and awkward to administer because it could not be dissolved in drinks.

Physicians quickly found ways round these difficulties. It was reported, for example, that 'a solution may be obtained by adding a few drops of acetic acid. It may also be rubbed up with sugars and dispensed in powders.'[2] By 1899 heroin hydrochloride was being advertised as 'a white crystalline powder easily soluble in water'.[3] The two main varieties of heroin were therefore both in currency by the end of the nineteenth century.

The chemical differences between heroin base and heroin hydrochloride are critical to the ways they have been used. A little chemistry will be necessary to explain their different properties. As heroin base is pure diamorphine, it is relatively unstable. It is soluble in fat and alcohol, but not in water. It is more volatile and has a lower melting point. It is therefore suitable for smoking. Heroin hydrochloride is a diamorphine salt: a compound produced by reacting diamorphine with an acid, in this case hydrochloric acid. It is soluble in water, not in alcohol or fat. It has a high melting point and tends to decompose with heat rather than turn into vapour. It is not much good for smoking, but because of its solubility in water it is good for injecting. It can also be sniffed in through the nose, where it dissolves easily in the mucous secretions coating the blood-rich olfactory membranes.

Although the two preparations lend themselves to different methods of consumption, once they are in the body their mode of action is identical. Heroin hydrochloride is in fact rapidly broken down to heroin base. After this, the solubility of heroin base in fat turns out to be very important in helping it penetrate the brain. For the most part, substances do not pass freely from the blood into the brain. They are prevented by a number of physiological defences which are collectively called the 'blood/brain barrier'. Its purpose is to prevent toxic confusion and brain damage when poisons are accidentally eaten. Substances that are highly fat-soluble find it much easier to cross this barrier. Heroin passes over with particular ease, leading to high concentration in the brain very soon after consumption. It is this sudden surge in brain concentration of the drug that is responsible for the characteristic heroin 'rush', so prized by its acolytes.

At the end of the nineteenth century, heroin was mostly taken by mouth and the majority of heroin preparations came from normal pharmaceutical sources. Taking heroin by mouth is not the best way, because most of it gets broken down to morphine during the process of digestion. For this reason, addicts very rarely take it this way. In the early days, however, heroin was mostly used as a cough medicine and as a treatment for tuberculosis. A number of syrups and tablets were sold, with various additives to improve its palatability or to increase its effectiveness in dealing with respiratory complaints.

Glyco-heroin was one popular cough mixture, advertised as 'suiting the palate of the most discerning adult or the most capricious child'. In 1902, Parke Davis announced some new tablets which disintegrated easily in water and were comprised of terpin (an expectorant) and heroin, the whole coated with chocolate.[4] Doctors could also prescribe more complex cocktails such as *Syrup Herophosphides*, consisting of hypophosphates of iron and manganese, lime, quinine, strychnine and heroin.[5] It is probable that this type of preparation influenced the ingredients in later illicit heroin recipes. *Syrup of Tolu and Heroin* was an exotic mixture, which acted as a sedative expectorant and would be welcomed by many flu sufferers today. In each fluid ounce, there were 20 mg heroin and 150 mg cannabis, along with tartar emetic, chloroform and syrup of tolu.[6] Heroin cough mixtures remained popular home remedies, until they mostly vanished as a result of restrictive legislation. However, in Britain up until 1949, the official British pharmaceutical catalogue, the Pharmacopoeia, still contained preparations such as an elixir of heroin and terpin, made up with cherry water.[7]

Pill divans and dragon-chasing

Heroin tablets were also used to some extent as a cure for morphine and opium dependence. For the most part, physicians warned against this practice, realising that heroin was at least as addictive as other opiates. Nonetheless, there was little control anywhere of medicines sold across the counter at the turn of the last century. In the United States, 'cures' for opium and morphine dependence were sold in drugstores and by mail order. Many of these tablets contained opiates themselves and therefore were miraculously successful in curtailing drug craving. The only snag was that the sufferer had to keep taking more and more of the cure![8] It is claimed that an American charitable society, the Society of St James, contemplated mounting a campaign to supply free doses of heroin through the mail to morphine addicts who wanted to give up their habit.[9]

Heroin pills became very popular in China and Hong Kong. They were used as a general tonic, but also particularly as 'anti-opium medicine' during the various government crackdowns on opium smoking. The first government seizures of these tablets occurred in

1921, but it is likely that by this time their use was widespread. They were usually pink and contained heroin, caffeine, strychnine and quinine, often flavoured with rose water. Probably this mixture owed something to earlier cough medicine cocktails, but interestingly these ingredients continue to feature in illicit heroin mixtures up until the present day.

Many unofficial chemists joined in the business. Pill-takers compared the merits of Golden Dragon, Tiger, Fairy Horse and countless other brands, each made with slightly different constituents. The pills were stridently advertised. A typical leaflet proudly proclaimed:

> It is hereby announced that I have studied medicine for over ten years and have spent several years of painstaking work in inventing CHAN LENG TEN one of the most efficacious of medicines. It is unanimously applauded and said to be the best medicine in the world.

Faced with these claims, it is not surprising that they became immensely popular. Over ten tons of heroin was used to make these pills in 1923 alone.

Opium smokers soon discovered that these pills could replace opium at a cheaper price. China has a long tradition of opium smoking. It is not surprising therefore that people started trying to smoke the heroin pills. Porcelain pipes were constructed, sometimes by snapping the spout off wine jugs, and placing the pill on the hole where the spout would have entered the jug. A bamboo pipe would be inserted into the neck of the jug, and the pipe sucked while an oil lamp was held to the pill. Usually ten to twenty pills would be smoked in a row, with heavy smokers taking up to 500 tablets a day. Many casual opiate takers preferred smoking pills to opium. They found it cleaner and quicker. It was also less likely to lead to constipation, which is the perennial curse of the opiate addict. Twenty cents' worth of pills was about the equivalent of fifty cents' worth of opium. It was therefore preferred by poorer people, who could not afford opium. 'Pill divans' began to replace the old opium dens.

At first the authorities were baffled by their seizures of pills. Government tests showed that no heroin at all was present in the smoke from the pills. It was assumed that the users were getting high on the caffeine in the pills rather than the heroin. However, when the tests were repeated with more sensitive equipment, it was discovered that a certain small amount of heroin could be extracted by this process.[10, 11] It was not enough to feed a serious habit, but it was sufficient for moderate users, provided enough pills were smoked.[12]

The habit continued to increase until the outbreak of World War II. In 1936 the Hong Kong government reported that they had seized over 180 million tablets and that 'the traffic in diacetylmorphine pills has increased to such an extent as to overshadow the whole drug situation in Hong Kong'. At about this time, the pills appeared briefly in the United States and seizures were made in Chicago, Detroit and New York. However, the habit never caught on in America and had disappeared by the war.[13] In Hong Kong, however, the pills were still being made according to exactly the same formula in 1974, but now mainly to supply a small group of ageing pill addicts.[14] For younger users, the technology of heroin smoking had moved on and become more sophisticated.

In 1939 stricter laws were passed in Hong Kong against pill smoking. During World War II, it was to some extent replaced by a new craze, called 'ack-ack' smoking. This involved dipping a cigarette in heroin, so that the tip was covered. The user then leant back with his face upwards, so that the heroin would not fall off. Smoking quickly, he would release rapid puffs of smoke towards the ceiling, in the process giving a fair imitation of an anti-aircraft gun.[15]

It was only in the early 1950s that 'chasing the dragon' was first noted in Hong Kong. This is a difficult technique, but one that has since spread halfway round the world. In the early days, chasers used heroin hydrochloride with four times the quantity of what was called 'base powder' or 'daai fan'. This consisted of a barbiturate sleeping powder. Lines of heroin and base powder were placed on creased tin foil and the foil was heated with a cigarette lighter or an oil lamp. The art of chasing is to make the heroin run smoothly over the foil, and to vaporise rather than let it burn and decompose. The smoker chases the vapour round the foil, and inhales it through a thin tube. If he is not very skilled, he may use a larger container such as an empty matchbox to inhale the smoke. It was then called 'playing the mouth-organ'.[16]

Chasing the dragon is not easy. It requires considerable dexterity to move the foil and tube effectively, and to apply heat at exactly the right temperature. Once mastered, however, it enables heroin to be smoked quickly and efficiently. Heroin is vaporised and inhaled at least ten times more efficiently, when compared with pill-smoking. It is therefore adequate for an addict with a serious habit. There is also less chance of detection, since there is no longer any need for pipes or other bulky equipment. For this reason, it spread quickly after the war when the governments in Hong Kong and China were pursuing opiate addicts with increased severity.

We explained that heroin hydrochloride is not good for smoking. However, its smokability is definitely improved by adding barbiturate powder. Laboratory experiments have shown that the amount of heroin vaporised is greatly increased when it is mixed with barbiturate.[17] The improvement is even greater with the addition of caffeine. The best combination of all is a mixture of caffeine and heroin base. It is not known how these discoveries were made. Caffeine was present in the heroin pills, but it was there even before the pills started to be smoked. It was probably a chance discovery that caffeine helped the vaporisation of heroin.

Before long, the barbiturate/heroin mixture for smoking was replaced by a powder named Chinese No. 3. Interestingly, the ingredients of this powder were almost exactly the same as the ingredients of the heroin pills, namely heroin, caffeine, strychnine and quinine, usually diluted with lactose. This is a good smoking mixture, but some of the ingredients are puzzling. The caffeine clearly helped the process of heroin vaporisation, but strychnine had the opposite effect. Quinine does not help or hinder. The composition of the mixture probably owes as much to conservatism in the heroin cooks and consumers as it does to chemical innovation. The addition of strychnine and quinine was an idea inherited from earlier times, when heroin was a cough medicine and general tonic.

Chinese No. 3 first appeared in Europe in 1973, to the puzzlement of police scientists. It was reported that heroin consisting of grey or pink-brown granules had been seized in Amsterdam. On analysis it contained 50 to 70 per cent heroin, 30 to 45 per cent caffeine and 0.5 to 10 per cent strychnine. Letters of enquiry were sent to fourteen laboratories worldwide, but thirteen were equally puzzled. Only the laboratory in Hong Kong was able to provide the helpful information that this type of heroin was used for smoking. This news was not passed on to the Dutch addicts, who continued to inject it. Scientists were worried that addicts might be poisoning themselves with strychnine, but analysis revealed that the amount absorbed was well below a dangerous dose.[18]

Chasing the dragon with Chinese No. 3 slowly spread around the East. It reached Thailand, Singapore and Malaysia in the 1970s, and India and Pakistan in the 1980s. Chasing did not really catch on in Europe until the early 1980s. From about 1975 a new type of heroin became available in Europe, mostly stemming from Iran. This heroin was a soft, fine powder, beige to dark in colour and with a characteristic odour. It was often called 'brown sugar'. It consisted of 70 to 80 per cent heroin base, with added caffeine. As such, it was ideally suited to smoking. Later on, as a result of political developments in South-West Asia, it was replaced by a very similar powder stemming from Pakistan, but probably produced by the same manufacturers.[19] Heroin prices fell by 25 per cent, but purity remained the same. By the late 1980s this heroin was being smoked in England, Spain, Holland and Italy.[20]

The same type of heroin still predominates in Europe today, although now it mostly comes from Afghanistan. Although it is smoking heroin, many users prefer to take it by injection. Because it is heroin base, it does not dissolve in water. For this reason, an acid has to be added to convert it into a salt, before it can be dissolved and drawn into the syringe. Most commonly, citric acid is used. This is usually obtained from a chemist or a needle exchange facility, but sometimes takes the form of lemon juice. Alternatively acetic acid may be used, in the form of vinegar. The process is not perfect, and usually some of the drug remains undissolved. It is reckoned that a user will usually extract the equivalent of 200 mg pharmaceutical heroin from a gram of this type of street heroin; in other words, about 20 per cent. This is partly because the heroin is usually sold with a purity of about 40 per cent. On top of this, a lot of heroin is lost in the process of dissolving, filtering and drawing up the liquid into the syringe.

Although users have worked out that heroin base will dissolve in water when converted to a salt, they have not discovered, or have not made use of the knowledge, that it dissolves well in alcohol. There are occasional reports of people injecting alcohol. Recently, tales circulated of sturdy Geordies injecting themselves with a local ale named Newcastle Brown. We are unaware yet of addicts injecting themselves with heroin dissolved in vodka or other strong spirits. Or perhaps those who have tried it have not survived to pass on the technique.

Happiness is a warm gun

Heroin use in the United States has been different from the start. Heroin hydrochloride has been used and it has been taken by snorting and injecting, often at low purity. Initially, pharmaceutical grade heroin was easily available from local drug stores. It quickly took over from opium, partly as a result of police pressure on opium dens. As a doctor remarked at the time,

It was cheap, it demanded neither layout nor hypodermic syringe, and could be taken for a long time without disturbing the health. It stopped the craving without diminishing working capacity to a degree which would prevent the earning of money to buy the drug, and last, but not least, as it is sniffed through the nose on a 'quill', the addict could take it without much fear of being interfered with.[21]

The quill was a straw, or a rolled up piece of paper. It is likely that this method of use was suggested by the similar method of taking cocaine, which was widely used in the United States at the turn of the last century.

Between about 1920 and 1950, legal pressure on drug takers and traffickers was severe and unremitting. The main result was a steep fall in the purity of heroin. It was reckoned that at times street heroin fell to a purity level of about 5 per cent. In consequence, users started to inject the drug. Injection is the best way to ensure that all the drug gets into your body and you get the maximum amount of 'bangs for your buck'.

At first, the method of injection was hypodermic: a skin-fold was raised and the drug was injected just under the skin using a hypodermic syringe. This type of injection had been popular since the Civil War and had been particularly used for administering morphine. The practice had led to widespread morphine dependence or 'morphino-mania' and to much concern in the medical profession. At this date, intravenous injection was only rarely used in medical practice, mostly for the treatment of crises such as morphine overdoses. Rather than injecting straight through the skin into the vein, the doctor would first expose the vein by cutting down through the overlying tissues with a scalpel.

In this climate, addicts tried to avoid veins when they injected through fear of a possible lethal reaction. It is uncertain who it was who discovered that intravenous (IV) injection was not inevitably fatal and, moreover, that it brought with it a new experience: the quasi-orgasmic heroin 'rush'. The rush depends on a very rapid rise in brain heroin concentration, which only occurs after IV injection. It is likely that it was discovered independently by a number of users during the 1920s.

The IV method of injection is first mentioned in the United States in 1925. There are two separate accounts of addicts who hit the vein by mistake and became very frightened. They then discovered that the experience was pleasant and started to tell their friends. The earliest of these accounts came from Terre Haute, Indiana, which can perhaps therefore claim the title of the home of IV drug abuse. Egypt could also put in a strong claim. Injecting was recorded in Cairo in 1925 and was later used by seamen. The practice spread down the Egyptian coast. It appears to have died out there by 1929, following an outbreak of sub-tertian malaria which was probably spread as a result of shared needles and syringes.[22]

O'Donnell and Jones have considered the question as to why IV injection only appeared a hundred years after the invention of the hypodermic syringe. They argue that IV injection would not have been possible for morphinomaniacs in the previous century, because they were using pure pharmaceutical morphine. If they had hit their veins by accident, it would have led to overdose and no desire among survivors to repeat the experiment. Moreover, most of the morphine addicts had acquired their addiction as a result of medical treatment. They would not have had the same reckless approach to experimentation as the 'kicks' addicts of the 1920s. In order for IV drug use to appear, there were a number of requirements: low drug purity, easy availability of needles and syringes, and lots of addicts who were chasing pleasure rather than medical treatment. This combination of circumstances first appeared in the United States between 1920 and 1925, and there was therefore a high likelihood that IV injecting would emerge at this time.[23]

This hypothesis is persuasive. Certainly, the practice spread quite quickly after discovery. Although it probably started among white users from the South, it spread most quickly among blacks, probably because it was the most economical way to take heroin. By 1935, 42 per cent of both black and white admissions to a government drug hospital were taking heroin intravenously. By 1940, 86 per cent of blacks were injecting and by 1950 it was 94 per cent, compared with 67 per cent of whites. Males were more likely to inject into the vein, whereas women on the whole continued to inject under the skin.[23] A characteristic of American injecting at this time was the use of the eye-dropper. Because syringes were hard to obtain, addicts created their own apparatus, usually with the rubber squeezers designed for administering eye-drops.

The United States also had its episodes of malaria spread by heroin injecting, an alarming precursor of the later epidemics of AIDS and hepatitis. There was an outbreak of malaria in New York City in 1933.[24] A more discrete episode occurred when some men on a fishing party shared shots from one eye-dropper, making up their dose with swamp water in a single tin cup.[25]

It has been argued that quinine is added to heroin to act against malaria. This is unlikely. Quinine is a traditional treatment for malaria but, as we have seen, it was used in heroin mixtures well before any fears of needle-borne malaria occurred. The most likely reason for its persistence in mixtures is that its bitter taste gives the impression of greater strength to users trying to assess the strength of the drug by preliminary tasting.

Snorting and injecting have remained the predominant methods of heroin use in the United States and also in Canada. Smoking is rare or non-existent, except recently on the West Coast near Mexico. The reason for this difference from the Asian experience has often been debated. It has been pointed out that Americans have had a long love affair with injecting, going back to morphine injection in the Civil War. Some have claimed fancifully that the American love of technology attracts them to the mechanical apparatus of injecting, rather than the low-tech smooth and gentle process of smoking. Samples of smoking heroin have on occasions been seized in America, but it has never enjoyed any consistent market penetration.[26] Some have argued that it does not accord with American psychology. Injecting is yang, smoking is yin: the Americans are a yang people.

This argument is dubious. In the early days opium smoking achieved a certain localised popularity in the US, particularly on the West Coast, before it was suppressed. But unlike Hong Kong, opium smoking was suppressed quickly and effectively, so there was no time for alternative smoking technologies to evolve. Instead of heroin pills, which contained caffeine and were therefore somewhat smokable, the only alternative in the United States was pharmaceutical heroin hydrochloride, which remained widely available for some years after opium all but disappeared. This ensured a transfer of most addicts to a form of heroin that was not smokable. Combined with an injecting tradition, these developments led almost inevitably to an endemic pattern of intravenous use. Generally speaking, it is not usual for addicts to transfer from injecting to smoking, even in places such as the UK where both practices are found together. Once injecting was established, it was unlikely that consignments of smoking heroin would have made much impact, even if users knew what to do with it. The different traditions in East and West are more likely to be due to history rather than national psychology. This view is supported by the growing popularity of heroin injection in China and other Asian countries during the last decade.

Whatever the explanation, injecting became an essential part of American heroin culture. Writer and heroin user Anna Kavan described the close relationship between the user and their injecting equipment in her autobiographical story about Julia and her 'bazooka':

Julia likes the doctor as soon as she meets him. He is under-standing and kind like the father she has imagined but never known. He does not want to take her syringe away. He says, 'You've used it for years already and you're none the worse. In fact you'd be far worse off without it.'[27]

Happiness is indeed a warm gun.

What's in a recipe?

Experts can identify different brands of heroin through their appear-ance and chemical composition. Chinese No. 3 was grey and granular, whereas Chinese No. 4 was white and crystalline. Indian heroin was dirty white, Pakistani beige and Syrian orange-brown. Penang Pink and Mexican Black Tar were the colours you would expect from their names. A form of smoking heroin from Hong Kong was dyed red and hence named Red Chicken.

When analysing composition, chemists divide what they find into three categories and call them, somewhat dryly, impurities, diluents and adulterants. Connoisseurs might prefer to call the last two mixers and flavours. Impurities are a result of the manufacturing process, and normally indicate some lack of efficiency in extracting morphine from opium and converting the morphine to heroin. They do not occur in pharmaceutical heroin. Typical impurities are acetylcodeine, papaverine and meconic acid.[28] Acetylcodeine concentration is particularly useful in determining the origin of a sample of heroin, because different regions and manufacturers have different 'acetylcodeine signatures'.[29] Acetylcodeine also forms the basis of a useful test for discovering whether addicts prescribed heroin are supplementing their supplies with additional purchased street heroin. Pharmaceutical heroin contains no acetylcodeine, so if it appears in the urine, it must have come from an illicit source.

Diluents are 'cutting agents', substances added by the manufacturer or dealer to add bulk through the process of 'cutting'. Contrary to general belief, cutting agents are usually safe and predictable.[30] Seized samples of heroin remain remarkably constant in different regions, both in terms of composition and of purity. It is not true that heroin is often made up with bizarre and dangerous ingredients such as bleach or worming powders. Common cutting agents are mannitol, lactose and powdered sugar. These are all relatively neutral agents that have little or no physiological effect in the quantities normally absorbed. They also do not contribute to the taste of the product.

Adulterants, on the other hand, are added on purpose to increase the effect or alter the taste. They give a brand of heroin its particular flavour and feel. Many of these ingredients go back to the beginning of the last century and are passed down from cook to cook in the same way that a recipe for fruitcake might be passed down through the generations. Common adulterants include quinine, which gives a bitter taste, and procaine, which has a local anaesthetic effect helpful for injectors. Caffeine and barbiturates help smokers achieve vaporisation while smoking. Methadone and amphetamine have been found on occasions, providing an extra kick.[31]

Although there are many different brands of heroin, it remains the case that there are two main types into which they can nearly all be categorised. First, there is a variety that is about 80 to 90 per cent pure heroin hydrochloride and is intended principally for injection. This is equivalent to Chinese No. 4. This is the major variety found today in South-East Asia, Australia and the United States. In Asia and Australia, this heroin comes almost entirely from the Golden Triangle between Thailand and Myanmar. American heroin was supplied from both Mexico and Asia, but more and more now comes from other Latin American countries, such as Peru and Colombia, as the cocaine barons start to diversify.

The second variety consists of heroin base, about 65 per cent pure originally. This is intended principally for smoking, although it is also often injected. This is the predominant variety in Europe and Russia. It comes almost entirely from Afghanistan. Both varieties are often cut down locally into lower purities, but not always. In Australia, for example, most street heroin is at least 85 per cent pure, which is one reason why Australian addicts often die young.

Recently, a black, gummy form of heroin has appeared in the United States. Called Mexican Black, it probably derives from unskilled producers in Chiapas province of Mexico. This may be a result of successful government suppression of traditional Mexican production networks. Mexican Black is impure heroin base and therefore not suitable for injecting. Unfortunately, American users are accustomed to the needle and as a result many have contracted nasty infections after injection, including a disease called botulism which is frequently fatal. More successfully, Mexican Black is sometimes dissolved in acetone and then cut down with lactose. This produces a mixture better adapted for the American market.

Occasionally, when there is a sudden change in routes of production and distribution, rogue forms of heroin like Mexican Black appear on the market. As a general rule, however, heroin distribution has become increasingly globalised. Big producers, often with unofficial or official government backing, have come to dominate the market and the varieties of heroin worldwide are less than there used to be. The time has perhaps come for a 'real heroin' campaign to rescue vanishing regional recipes!

Does he still take brown sugar?

In some countries, heroin is predominantly taken in one manner, for example smoked in cigarettes in Pakistan or injected in Australia. In other countries, two or more methods of use coexist. In Britain, smoking and injecting are equally common, whereas in the United States the choice is mostly between injecting and snorting. Health workers are interested in how people choose their route of use, and whether they tend to stick to one route or change between them. They want to know whether they can persuade people to move away from injecting to a safer route like snorting or smoking. If people often make this type of transition, then campaigns against injecting have a better chance of success.

It appears that choice of route often depends on previous experience with other drugs. Familiarity with cocaine may have led to heroin snorting in New York. Londoners stemming from the West Indies have a strong tradition of cannabis smoking. They are more likely than white users to smoke rather than inject heroin. In North-West England, amphetamine injection was widespread before heroin arrived. It was natural therefore that many new heroin users quickly moved into injecting. Women are more likely than men to snort or smoke.

Once a route is chosen, it remains fairly steady. People tend to see themselves as smokers, sniffers or injectors. In one study in South London, it was found that out of 408 users, 54 per cent were injectors and 44 per cent chasers. Only a third of these had changed route once in their life and very few had changed route twice. Many users remained smokers throughout their heroin career. There is some risk of people moving from smoking to injecting, but changes also occur in the other direction. A move from smoking to injecting is about twice as likely as a move from injecting to smoking.[32] These figures do give some support to the idea that it is worth trying to move people towards smoking, and they also provide hope that, if such a move were made, many users would stick to smoking rather than inevitably reverting to the needle.

However, they also indicate how important it is to persuade people not to start injecting in the first place. Nearly all the health risks attached to heroin derive from the practice of injecting. It is very difficult to avoid Hepatitis C infection if you inject, and there are also the risks of Hepatitis B, AIDS, abscesses and thrombosis, and septicaemia. The majority of users who start injecting continue to do so throughout their career. Public health agencies are beginning to realise that their advertising energies should be directed not so much against using heroin, but against injecting heroin.

High-tech heroin – the horse gallops on

There has been considerable evolution in modes of heroin use over the last century, and an ongoing interaction between mode of consumption and heroin formulation. The heroin chemists have made strenuous efforts to adapt their preparations to the popular method of use. At the same time, the types of heroin available have had an effect on patterns of consumption. New techniques have gradually diffused across national borders and between ethnic groups. Nonetheless, there remains considerable regional variety.

Heroin technology is certain to continue evolving. In historical terms, it is a very recent arrival in the world of intoxicants. Compared with alcohol, present use is about as advanced as home-fermented maize beer. As we will describe in the final chapter, there are a number of technological advances in the pipeline which are likely to change the way heroin is taken. These include smart needles, in-dwelling pumps, compressed-gas powder guns and ultrasound-operated skin pads. Moreover, advances in chemistry will allow more rapid and efficient testing of mixtures and recipes.

Recently, the Swiss and Dutch have mounted some research trials of heroin prescription to heroin addicts. The outcome of these trials will be described in Chapter 8. With typical thoroughness, the Swiss considered many possible methods of heroin consumption before deciding to base their trial mostly around injection. During the preliminary studies, they considered heroin aerosol sprays, laced herbal tobacco cigarettes and even heroin suppositories.[33] Meanwhile, the Dutch developed for their trial a tablet of heroin and caffeine, heated on a small electric coil.

Once the big chemists get involved, the Shanghai mastercooks may have to step aside. Who knows what techniques and what varieties of heroin the next hundred years may bring?

Notes

1 'Analytical records – heroin', *Lancet* (3 December 1898): 1,486.
2 Manges, M. (1899) 'The treatment of coughs with heroin', *New York Medical Journal* 68: 768–70.
3 'Analytical records', *Lancet* (6 May 1899): 1,235.
4 'New preparations received', *British Medical Journal* (4 January 1902): 28.
5 'Analytical records', *Lancet* (18 May 1901): 1,410.
6 'Analytical records', *Lancet* (24 December 1904): 1,791.
7 'Heroin in the official pharmacopoeia', *Bulletin on Narcotics* 5 (1953): 19.
8 Musto, D.F. (1999) *The American Disease: Origins of Narcotic Control*, New York: Oxford University Press.
9 Latimer, D. and Goldberg, J. (1981) *Flowers in the Blood. The Story of Opium*, New York: Franklin Watts.
10 Ito, R. (1936) 'Amount of effective component which passes into smoke when heroin is smoked', *Journal of Oriental Medicine* 24: 76–8.
11 Adams, E.W. (1937) *Drug Addiction*, Oxford: Oxford University Press.
12 'The mysterious heroin pills for smoking', *Bulletin on Narcotics* 5 (1953): 54–9.
13 Valaer, P. (1935) 'The red pill or the opium substitute', *American Journal of Pharmacy* 107: 199–207.
14 Confidential report of the Royal Hong Kong Police Narcotics Bureau (1973) *Heroin Manufacture in Hong Kong* (September).
15 Mo, B.P. and Way, E.L. (1966) 'An assessment of inhalation as a mode of administration of heroin by addicts', *Journal of Pharmacology and Experimental Therapeutics* 154: 142–51.
16 Gruhzit, C.G. (1958) 'Pharmacological investigation and evaluation of the effects of combined barbiturate and heroin inhalation by addicts', *Bulletin on Narcotics* 10: 8–11.
17 Huizer, H. (1987) 'Analytical studies on illicit heroin. V. Efficacy of volatilisation during heroin smoking', *Pharmaceutish Weekblad (Scientific Edition)* 9: 203–11.
18 Eskes, D. and Brown, J.K. (1975) 'Heroin–caffeine–strychnine mixtures – where and why?', *Bulletin on Narcotics* 27: 67–9.
19 O'Neil, P., Baker, P.B. and Gough, T.A. (1984) 'Illicitly imported heroin products: some physical and chemical features indicative of their origin', *Journal of Forensic Sciences* 29: 89–92.
20 Strang, J., Griffiths, P. and Gossop, M. (1997) 'Heroin smoking by "chasing the dragon": origins and history', *Addiction* 92: 673–83.
21 Bailey, P. (1916) 'The heroin habit', *New Republic* 6: 314–16.
22 Biggam, A.G., Arafa, M.A. and Ragab, A.F. (1932) 'Heroin addiction in Egypt and its treatment during the withdrawal period', *Lancet* 1: 922–7.
23 O'Donnell, J.A. and Jones, J.P. (1968) 'Diffusion of the intravenous technique among narcotic addicts in the United States', *Journal of Health and Social Behaviour* 9: 121–30.
24 Helpern, M. (1934) 'Malaria among drug addicts in New York City', *Public Health Reports, Washington* 49: 421.
25 Himmelsbach, C.K. (1933) 'Malaria in narcotic addicts', *Public Health Reports, Washington* 48: 1,465.
26 Kalant, H. (1997) 'Supply reduction v. demand reduction: the uses of history', *Addiction* 92: 689–90.

27 Kavan, Anna (1970) *Julia and the Bazooka*, London: Peter Owen.
28 O'Neil, P., Phillips, G.F. and Gough, T.A. (1985) 'The detection and characterisation of controlled drugs imported into the UK', *Bulletin on Narcotics* 37: 17–32.
29 Narayanaswami, K. (1985) 'Parameters for determining the origin of illicit heroin samples', *Bulletin on Narcotics* 37: 49–62.
30 Coomber, R. (1997) 'Vim in the veins – fantasy or fact? The adulteration of illicit drugs', *Addiction Research* 5: 195–212.
31 'The analysis of heroin', *Bulletin on Narcotics* 5 (1953): 27–34.
32 Griffiths, P., Gossop, M., Powis, B. and Strang, J. (1994) 'Transitions in patterns of heroin administration: a study of heroin chasers and heroin injectors', *Addiction* 89: 301–9.
33 Uchtenhagen, A. *et al.* (1999) *Prescription of Narcotics for Heroin Addicts. Main results of the Swiss National Cohort Study*, Basle: Karger.

3 *How to X-ray a camel*
The spread of heroin and
attempts at control

Heroin first saw the light of day a century and a quarter ago in a laboratory near Paddington Station in London. Since then it has spread across the world in fits and starts, temporarily held up here or blocked there, but pushing on with an urgency that has eventually overcome all obstacles. There still remain places, such as Africa and South America, where its use is rare, but nobody expects it to stay that way for long. All indications are that heroin will be available across the whole globe by 2010. Moreover, in countries where it is already easily obtained, the tendency over recent years has been for purity to increase and prices to fall.

The international effort to control its spread has not been successful, in spite of temporary triumphs. Many good people have done their best, but fingers in the dyke have not been enough. It is a reasonable guess that before long heroin control will form a footnote in history, like previous efforts to check the spread of coffee and alcohol. This is no cause for celebration, but perhaps when this failure is recognised the huge amount of money spent on the effort can be diverted to more worthwhile tasks. These would include promoting abstinence, encouraging moderate use for those who can't abstain and treating the severely dependent.

At first it seemed that controls would be successful. The history can be neatly divided into three periods. Before World War I heroin use was largely unregulated. Between the wars, laws were passed and conventions were agreed, with considerable success. Since the end of World War II increasingly powerful criminal organisations have learnt how to side-step international controls, often with the support of corrupt governments. Unfortunately memories of earlier successes have persuaded some policy-makers that a 'war on drugs' can still be won. We are now perhaps entering a fourth phase in which this metaphorical war has itself got out of control and is causing much more harm than it attempts to prevent.

Early freedom and first concerns – the United States and China

During the first decade of the twentieth century, heroin was widely available in many countries, either by direct purchase or through a doctor's prescription. Heroin was not yet well known or popular among the public. There were already many opiate addicts, but morphine and opium were the principal drugs consumed. Morphine addiction was already widespread in the United States and Europe. In the States, in particular, morphine- and cocaine-containing compounds had been dispensed freely by drugstores without any control. It is reckoned that opiate dependence was as prevalent in the States in 1870 as it was in 1970, but instead of being confined to socially marginal groups it was found principally among the middle classes, particularly women. Large quantities of opium were imported into the States for the manufacture of morphine. Although morphine use in Europe was also common, it was much less so than in the States. For example, during the first decade of the century, one hundred times as much opium was imported into the States as into Austro-Hungary, even though the population was only twice as large.[1]

In many countries in the East, opium itself was smoked and it was socially acceptable and legal. Opium smoking first arrived in the United States with the Chinese. Between 1852 and 1870, 70,000 Chinese came to the United States to work on the railroads and in the gold mines, and many of these workers smoked opium to relax after a hard day's work. The practice spread to a limited extent among the local population, particularly on the West Coast, and in the 'tenderloin' districts of cities like San Francisco. At the same time, morphine was becoming popular in China, thanks to the entrepreneurial activity of European pharmaceutical firms.

Cultures are relatively happy with their own drugs but suspicious of those used by aliens. It is an irony typical of the history of drug use that American legislators began to see opium as a dangerous Oriental custom that was threatening the morality of their people, at the same time as aspiring Chinese nationalists yearned to throw off the degrading tyranny of foreign capitalism and along with it the enslavement of their people through drugs peddled by Western pharmacists. It was this symmetrical attitude in the two countries that led in time to the suppression of opium and morphine, and the eventual triumph of heroin.

State laws against opium use were first enacted on the West Coast of America in 1875, but action taken under these laws was often greeted with some incredulity.[2] Some state anti-morphine laws were passed, but in effect there was little control on the supply of heroin and morphine in drugstores until the Pure Food and Drug Act of 1906. Many proprietary medicines not only contained significant quantities of morphine, cocaine and heroin but also provided consumers with no indication of what they contained.[3]

The Pure Food and Drug Act required no more than accurate labelling of drugs and recording of sales, but it was still widely resisted. Nonetheless, an impetus had developed towards the control of drug dependence. There was growing concern about the extent of morphine and opium addiction. There was also a mood for health and environmental legislation. This encompassed widespread laws against tobacco[4] and would also lead eventually to the Volstead Act of 1919, which initiated the era of alcohol prohibition. American colonial interests provided a further incentive. They had acquired the Philippines in 1895[5] and they were keen to obtain a share in the developing Chinese market, hitherto parcelled out among the older colonial powers.

In the Philippines, American administrators had come face to face with endemic opium smoking and felt obliged to respond. Elsewhere in Asia, opium smoking was widely permitted until after World War II. For example, in Malaysia the British government tolerated it under increasingly tight controls, while continuing to ensure a supply of income for the state. It was not banned altogether until 1945. Similarly, in Thailand, King Rama IV imposed high taxes on opium during the nineteenth century, but the sale of opium was not banned until 1958.[6] With hindsight it appears that this tolerance prevented the early encroachment of heroin. America decided to take a firmer line. It investigated the attitude of other colonial powers to opium, but concluded that the only effective laws were the strict ones 'enacted by Japan for the main part of the Empire, and for Formosa'.[7] Following this inquiry, Congress ordered a total ban on opiates in the Philippines, except for medicinal purposes.[8]

In China, resentment had been growing against the opium trade, which the government had been powerless to resist following defeat by the British in the Opium Wars. The spread of addiction had been one of the causes of unrest that had led to the Boxer Rising. Following suppression of the revolt, the failing imperial regime had begun to take stern action against local trafficking and was also looking for support in banning international trade. This pressure intensified after nationalist revolutionaries had finally toppled the Manchu Dynasty in 1911. American diplomats reasoned that if they could help China deal with its problem, they would thereby win access to lucrative new markets.

The wheel had turned full circle. The American movement that originally aimed to eradicate an oriental vice from America ended up supporting a Chinese movement to eradicate a Western vice from China.

If the Americans were going to take the lead in campaigning against the international opium trade, they had to show they were serious by passing internal legislation. In 1909 Congress passed a law forbidding the import of opium, except for medicinal purposes. Primarily this affected opium smokers in the local Chinese community, who could be seen as a soft target. There then followed a number of international conferences at American instigation, including the Shanghai Opium Commission Meetings of 1909 and the Hague International Conference on Opium of 1911–12. This led to the Hague Opium Convention of 1912, whereby each of the thirty-four signatory nations agreed to tighten domestic controls on the manufacture and distribution of opiates and cocaine, with a view to restricting their use to medical purposes. This led in time to various national laws, including the US Harrison Act of 1914 and the British Dangerous Drugs Act of 1920.

China and the United States had the largest opiate problems and therefore were most affected by this movement towards control. With the suppression of opium, heroin use began to increase in the States. For a period of several years it was easier to obtain than other opiates.

> Dope users who found that police surveillance made it very difficult to secure opium, morphine and cocaine soon learned that heroin could be easily obtained. No prescription is necessary. As a result they began using this drug, and the habit grew by leaps and bounds.[9]

This trend was strengthened by the passage of the Harrison Act.

> Opiate users, both old smokers and new recruits, have deserted for the most part all other habit-forming drugs for a new derivative of opium. This new drug, which was heroin, won an immediate and widespread popularity.[10]

Heroin became particularly popular in New York and, to a lesser extent, in other cities along the East Coast. This was probably because the pharmaceutical factories were clustered in New York.

What emerged was a phenomenon which has hugely influenced world attitudes to heroin. Opiate consumption was no longer the prerogative of middle-class ladies receiving nerve tonics from their doctors and druggists. It had been driven underground and was now used on the margins of society. Heroin addicts were 'in many instances members of gangs who congregate on street corners particularly at night, and make insulting remarks to people who pass'. When not engaged in robbery, they supported themselves by collecting scrap metal or 'junk'. These new-style 'junkies' were perceived to be as much a threat to society as anarchists.[11]

Moreover, the opiate used was seen as something strange and dangerous due to its unfamiliarity, even though pharmaceutically it was similar to morphine. A moral panic gripped the nation. Heroin was credited with huge powers and a bottomless capacity for evil. To some extent these exaggerated fears are still with us today. When America catches a cold, the world sneezes. American attitudes and prejudices have been hugely influential in shaping international policy.

Some saw heroin as a German device for depleting the war effort. Representative Henry Rainey claimed in Congress that '80,000 draftees had been rejected due to heroin addiction', although the true figure was nearer 3,000.[12] In 1919 the Mayor's Committee on Public Safety implicated heroin as being responsible for a series of anarchist bombings. In 1922 there were 260 murders in New York, compared to seventeen in London. Surely heroin was to blame; for as Dr Lambert observed later at Congressional hearings: 'Heroin destroys the sense of responsibility to the herd'. Not long afterwards Captain Richard T. Hobson, the eccentric self-publicist and anti-drugs campaigner, was warning all young mothers to check the food their children ate, to make sure it was not laced with heroin by unscrupulous dealers. He went further: 'in using any brand of face powder, it is a wise precaution to have a sample checked for heroin'.[13] The mood of the nation was summed up by the *New York Times*: 'ONE MILLION AMERICANS VICTIMS OF DRUG HABIT – Alarming increase of addicts called menace more dangerous than war'.[14]

Against this background, a hostile attitude to the medical treatment of drug misuse is understandable. The Harrison Act had not originally intended to ban the prescription of heroin or morphine for medical purposes. However, a series of court cases ruled against their prescription to addicts.[15] The authorities took steps to close clinics, such as those in New York and Shreveport, which were set up to maintain addicts on steady doses of opiates. In 1920 the police supported the American Medical Association (AMA) in adopting the resolution that 'heroin be eliminated from all medicinal preparations ... and that the importation, manufacture and sale of heroin should be prohibited in the US'. In 1922 it was estimated that 58 ounces of heroin had been prescribed throughout the whole of the United States, compared to 76,000 ounces used illegally on the streets of New York alone.[16] In 1924 an Act was passed in line with the AMA resolution and licit heroin virtually vanished. Not so illicit heroin; by 1928 a third of jail inmates were Harrison violators.[13]

In China, initial legislation was not so successful in reducing the flow of pharmaceutical opiates. Strict penalties against opium smoking encouraged Chinese users to move over to morphia injecting, as the apparatus was easier to use without detection. Between 1913 and 1920, huge quantities of morphine from British factories were imported into China, mostly by Japanese smugglers operating through Manchuria and Korea. In Manchuria itself, it appeared that the Japanese authorities encouraged the distribution of drugs 'as part of the policy for the peaceful penetration of Manchuria'. British embarrassment at this continuance of the opium trade by other means was initially tempered by reason of policy. A Foreign Office memo in 1917 shockingly advised that

> [the] prohibition of morphia exports would preclude a considerable number of Japanese from earning their living by poisoning the inhabitants of Manchuria and would therefore add fuel to the fire of Japanese irritation. In fact it would seem essentially a question to be postponed until the end of the war.[17]

Pushed by public pressure, Britain finally reached an agreement with Japan that export of morphine to Japan would only be allowed to manufacturers holding a licence from the Japanese government. This system of export licences was then gradually expanded through the League of Nations to include bilateral agreements between most countries involved in the narcotics trade. This system was strengthened in Britain by passage of the Dangerous Drugs Act of 1920. By 1923 British manufacturers had ceased to supply the illicit market. The last to be involved was T.E. Whiffen, which lost its manufacturing licence after prosecution for smuggling.[18]

Other European firms took over production, particularly firms in Germany, Holland, France and Switzerland. The Geneva Convention was signed in 1925 and implemented in 1928. It confirmed the system of licensed manufacture, and of export and import licences. It was the first to install an international regulatory body to control the trade. Nonetheless, there were many loopholes[19] and regulation remained weak. It is reckoned that in 1928 six tons of morphine products were sent from Europe to China. The Advisory Committee on Opium and

Other Dangerous Drugs pointed the finger of blame particularly at Germany, where (it was claimed) 18.6 tons of morphine products had been made in 1929, of which only 6 tons could conceivably be justified on medical grounds.[20] In spite of this wholesale contraband, it was not the sufferings of China that moved the international community to clamp down harder. The world had become inured to Chinese drug addiction. Much more frightening was sudden epidemic in a country which had been hitherto untainted.

The Egyptian outbreak and the international response

Apart from China and the United States, the one country that suffered an outbreak of heroin use between the wars was Egypt. Egypt's wretched experience had a powerful effect in increasing international anxieties and promoting the strengthening of controls. The problem apparently started with a handful of crooked pharmacists in Cairo selling white drugs to the expatriate community. A Greek chemist made a fortune selling cocaine, mostly to the social elite in 1926 and 1927. Shortly afterwards an Armenian chemist was recorded as selling over 600 kilograms of heroin in a year and it became clear that the drugs were spreading into the wider community. By 1929 almost one in four of all males aged between 20 and 40 were addicted to heroin.[21] At the same time an outbreak of subtertian malaria occurred, as a result of shared injecting equipment.[22] In certain districts labourers were being paid with heroin rather than money.

When this started in 1925, selling heroin and cocaine was perfectly legal. Though the laws and conventions were tightened, it still proved difficult for police to prosecute the guilty parties. Egypt was still subject to the ancient system of 'Capitulations'[23] whereby foreigners could not be prosecuted except through their own countries. The Bakar family in Alexandria was a notorious drug purveyor, but by claiming Italian nationality it secured the protection of the Italian consul-general and remained immune to prosecution.

Head of the Cairo police at the time was an Englishman named Thomas Russell. He had worked his way up the Egyptian Service under the British Protectorate, but was later to remain head of police for several years after Egyptian independence. His response to the crisis was energetic. He persuaded the government to pass new laws against the possession of drugs. He had been responsible for founding the Camel Corps back in 1906: this was now expanded to intercept smuggled drugs. Surveillance was also increased at border posts.

The drugs entered Egypt through various exotic supply routes. Much arrived concealed on the bodies of bogus monks and nuns or in the stomachs of camels. At that time, camels were still the major source of transport in Egypt. It is reckoned that over 30,000 camels a month passed through the quarantine station of Kantara alone, which posed a huge challenge to customs staff. Smugglers devised zinc cylinders, which were filled with heroin. When camels swallowed these cylinders, they were so designed that they stuck in their second stomachs and so were not digested, nor did they cause the camels any major harm until they were slaughtered for recovery of the heroin. X-ray machines were set up at quarantine centres to detect the cylinders, but it was only possible to film a small percentage of passing camels. Moreover, it was not long before smugglers started using plastic tubes which were transparent to X-rays.[24]

This type of border surveillance has never been successful in reducing drug imports. Where Russell was more effective was in infiltrating his agents into contraband supply. It became clear that these white drugs all stemmed from the large pharmaceutical companies in Europe, but were then passed on to contraband traders. A leading example was the Société Roessler et Compagnie, from Mulhouse in France, which in 1928 produced 4,349 kg of heroin, much of which ended up in Egypt. Other suppliers were the factories of Dr Hefti in Zurich and that of Dr Muller in Basle.[25] The system of import and export licences was easily evaded. As Russell wrote of Dr Hefti: 'Though morally reprehensible, his conduct was legally unimpeachable. His country's laws permitted him to manufacture moral and material poison in uncontrolled quantities.'

Armed with this evidence, Russell went in person to the League of Nations Opium Advisory Commission in 1930. His speech proved very influential.

> Before the introduction of these European poisons, there was no more healthy, hardworking and cheerful class of peasant in the world: today every village has its heroin victims, and they are the youth of the country. Can you picture your quiet little villages corrupted and poisoned with dope? You cannot, but I can, as I see it every day in Egypt. Gentlemen, I ask you: is it fair that Europe should thus pour its tons of poison into my country? Egypt is fighting to save itself, but cannot do so without your help.

His plea caused considerable shock and was reported by the press worldwide. It was a major factor in bringing about the Limitation

Convention of 1931, whose effect was to restrict the amount of heroin produced by factories in signatory countries to that which appeared reasonable for medical purposes. There was a move by many countries to abolish the manufacture of heroin altogether, but this proposal was eventually outvoted. Nonetheless, several countries did abolish heroin before the war, including the United States, Spain, Bulgaria, Costa Rica, Mexico, Greece and Poland.[16]

This Convention brought about the end of the contraband traffic in pharmaceutical heroin, with the exception of Japanese trade which was now sourced by new factories in Korea. It also helped Egypt to overcome its problem. By 1934 Russell was able to report back to the Commission that there had been a reduction of convicted addicts in Egypt from 5,681 in 1929 to 674 in 1933.[21]

Some success at last

Meanwhile, in the United States the Bureau of Narcotics was established as a separate entity in 1930. The first Commissioner was Harry Jacob Anslinger,[26] a man with a tough approach to addiction. For thirty-two years he led the American fight against drugs, relying on a simple principle:

> We intend to get the killer-pushers and their willing customers out of buying and selling drugs. The answer to the problem is simple – get rid of drugs, pushers and users. Period.[27]

The way you got rid of them was by locking them up, either in prison or later in reformatory 'drug farms' such as those established at Lexington in Kentucky and Fort Worth in Texas.[28] He was also tireless in pushing for international controls. He was one of the chief instigators of the Convention on Limitations, which proved an effective response to Egypt's epidemic. It must be said that his tactics had considerable success, although occasioning much misery for addicts. The number of American opiate addicts fell from 200,000 in 1924 to 20,000 in 1945.[29] Anslinger's activity provided a powerful example for later advocates of Nixon's 'War on Drugs'.

What happened to the old middle-class morphine addicts? It appears that physicians continued surreptitiously to prescribe for them and that the authorities connived at this practice. At a time when heroin addicts were suffering under oppressive legislation, officials reported that there were in a number of states 'from 200 to 400 or 500 elderly addicts maintained by physicians, against whom they had no idea of taking action'.[30] One such addict must have been Mrs Dubose, the cantankerous neighbour of Atticus in *To Kill a Mockingbird*. She won his children's admiration by managing to get off morphine before she died. It is significant that in this novel, set in the 1930s, no one expresses surprise that an old lady should be a morphine addict.[31] There may have been no recruitment of new therapeutic addicts, but there was certainly a large but diminishing cohort of old addicts right up to World War II.

A book on drug dependence written by a British physician affords a useful insight into world heroin use just before the outbreak of the war. He reckoned that about 1 per 1,000 US citizens were opiate addicts, with heroin being primarily used on the East Coast and morphine on the West. Similar figures were found in Canada, with heroin predominating. There was little heroin use in Europe. About 100 out of 700 British opiate addicts used heroin. In both Germany and Britain over 10 per cent of addicts were doctors. In Spain it was confined to 'convicted criminals in Madrid'. It was rare in France, 'except among demi-mondaines', and negligible in Romania and Switzerland. In Greece 'heroinists were mostly found in the army'. In Russia there was little drug addiction: it was 'confined to the medical profession, the Bohemian classes and the criminal stratum of society'. In Egypt a dramatic change had been wrought due to 'the splendid work of the Egyptian Central Narcotics Bureau under the devoted leadership of Russell Pasha'. Ethiopia 'shares with Newfoundland the felicity of having no narcotics problem'. Opium was still smoked, often under government licence, in many Asian countries. Burma had the highest number of opium users, with about 7 per 100 of the population. Heroin use was still very rare in these countries. In China there had recently been an increased consumption of white drugs, such as heroin, morphine and cocaine. This had prompted drastic measures: 'even decapitation may be the fate of the relapsed addict'. Ironically, 'the Japanese people are free from addiction owing to the strictness of their anti-narcotic laws'.[32]

Those who aimed to control the spread of heroin could congratulate themselves. Only Japanese drug production remained as a major problem and this would only be solved by military action.

Syndicates and gangs

During World War II, pharmaceutical heroin continued to be produced for consumption in Manchuria. Those who fell under its sway include the so-called 'Last Emperor of China', who was installed as a puppet ruler by the Japanese and kept in line by exploitation of his addiction. It continued to infiltrate the rest of China in spite of drastic attempts at control. In 1941 a law was passed that addicts would be shot if found injecting heroin powder or smoking pills. It was not this law that succeeded in stamping out the problem temporarily in China. The defeat of Japan led to closure of their pharmaceutical factories in Korea and suddenly turned off the major source of supply. In 1947 Mao Tse Tung defeated the Nationalist Army and set up the Chinese Republic, ushering in an era of unprecedented upheaval and social control. The Maoist revolution was mostly successful in eradicating drug misuse, but as we shall see this was only a temporary victory.

The immediate effect was the exodus of the drug syndicates from Shanghai to Hong Kong. Heroin use increased dramatically in Hong Kong, partly as a result of effective British laws against opium smoking. Hong Kong established itself as the main centre for heroin production in the East. At first, the trade was controlled by Shanghai triads, but later it was taken over by the Chiu Chau syndicate from Kwangtung. Hong Kong maintained its supremacy in the heroin trade, until police action in 1974 led to arrests and massive seizures. After this, most of the chemists and businessmen left for Thailand and Malaysia.[33]

The international fight against drugs passed in 1946 from the League of Nations to the newly formed United Nations. Pharmaceutical heroin was no longer available except under very tight control. Increasingly it was replaced by heroin manufactured in clandestine factories. During the late 1940s, illicit factories were discovered in Turkey, France, Mexico, Greece, Hong Kong and the United States. As the French reported:

> the discovery of the laboratory in Paris, following the discovery of a laboratory in Marseilles last year, show how easy it is to install an illicit laboratory for the conversion of morphine into heroin.

Turkey, China and later Hong Kong were the main sources of heroin at this time. Brown Mexican heroin was found in the United States and Canada, but almost disappeared after a clampdown by the authorities.[16] The main route for heroin entering the United States was from Turkey via France and Italy. This was the so-called 'French Connection'.[34] The way this functioned was in some ways typical of the post-war heroin business and gives a good indication of why well-meaning attempts at control have been doomed to failure.

The driving force behind the French Connection was a Sicilian American named Charlie 'Lucky' Luciano. He had made a fortune selling bootleg liquor during Prohibition and then achieved control of the American mafiosi following the gangster wars of 1930–31. Foreseeing the end of Prohibition, he diversified into heroin and pros- titution. He was finally imprisoned in 1936, but he continued to run his business from jail with the help of his associate, Meyer Lansky.

During the war, the US Navy was greatly concerned about the secu- rity of the New York waterfront, particularly after the troopship *Normandie* caught fire. Luciano was contacted in prison and, being a good American patriot, he agreed to use his network to ensure there were no further breaches of security. Not only that, but his contacts in Sicily later proved invaluable during General Patten's invasion. As a token of gratitude, he received an official pardon at the end of the war, but was deported to Italy.

Unfortunately, successful mobsters do not retire. By the end of the war, the supply of heroin to the United States had almost dried up. Only about 20,000 'survivors' were still using the drug and what they could get hold of was excessively weak. It is possible that had the supply remained as poor for a few years longer, the US heroin problem might have disappeared altogether. But it did not. Luciano set up a sweet factory in Italy and used this as a front to flood the States with heroin from Turkey.

The Criminal Intelligence Agency to the rescue

In 1947 the Office of Strategic Studies was restructured to form the Criminal Intelligence Agency (CIA). The Cold War was starting and a phobia of communism was pervading the Western democracies. Joseph McCarthy established the House Committee on Un-American Activities and began to persecute Americans with left-wing leanings. Alongside the Committee, President Truman envisaged the CIA forming a key element in the fight against communism. In the event, the CIA proved enthusiastic and ingenious. The security of the state and the struggle against the red menace was considered more impor- tant than the health of junkies. On many critical occasions, the CIA was happy to support drug dealers and producers if it gave them some strategic advantage over their enemies.

One of the CIA's first targets was to undermine communist parties in Europe. In order to subvert the French Communist Party, an alliance was formed with gangs from the Corsican underworld. Part of the deal was protection for the heroin production and distribution centres in Marseilles, which were controlled by the Corsicans and by Luciano. With the implicit support of the CIA and the French government, Marseilles remained the hub of the trade until the early 1970s. Large quantities of Lebanese and Turkish opium were processed there and shipped to the United States. By the time of Luciano's death in 1965, the number of heroin addicts in the US had increased to 150,000 and the problem had become endemic.

By 1970 the number had increased to 500,000. The huge increase since the war had been due to a combination of easy supplies and a ready market created in particular by the influx into the great conurbations of rural black families looking for work. In a generation, heroin became principally a drug used by black people and had become integrated into urban black culture. This development caused huge anxiety in middle-class America. A series of severe laws were passed, starting with the Boggs–Daniel Bill of 1956 that included provision of the death penalty for selling heroin to minors. A ten-year minimum and forty-year maximum spell of imprisonment was mandated for a second offence of possessing heroin or marijuana. All manufacture and importation of heroin was banned, and all hospitals had to surrender their remaining stocks. The rate of imprisonment for drug-related offences rose sharply. These measures were perhaps partly responsible for the reduction of US heroin use in the early 1970s, but undoubtedly the most important factor was the closure of the French Connection and the suppression of heroin production in Turkey as a result of UN pressure. By 1975 the number of US opiate addicts had fallen to 200,000.

Unfortunately, other sources of supply arose to fill the vacuum and, once again, the CIA was deeply implicated. In the early 1950s it had supported an unsuccessful Chinese nationalist attempt to invade South-West China. It later helped this army establish itself in Burma, in order to provide a buffer against Chinese infiltration of South-East Asia. It largely financed itself by opium production and for several years the Shan State of Burma was the largest opium producer in the world. It forms part of the Golden Triangle, which also includes neighbouring areas of Thailand and Cambodia, and which has remained to this day one of the world's major suppliers of heroin.

By 1960 the CIA was active in Laos as part of the struggle against North Vietnam. It helped establish a secret army of 30,000 Hmong tribesmen to fight against the Laotian communists. The Hmong were traditional opium producers. This was actively supported by the CIA as part of its friendship strategy, even to the extent of arranging transport of raw opium to processing laboratories in the Golden Triangle. Much of the heroin used by the American troops in Vietnam came from this source. The CIA therefore played a key role in fostering the production of heroin in South-East Asia.[29] This process was accelerated by the immigration of traders and chemists from Hong Kong following the British clampdown in 1974.

When Turkish supplies dried up, the successors of Luciano were quick to make contacts with the Golden Triangle. Asian heroin began to flow into the US and by 1980 the number of addicts had returned to 500,000, in spite of the strict legislation. With drugs of addiction, the laws of supply and demand tend to overpower the restraining activities of police and law courts. From this time on, there were no further heroin famines. It has been produced freely in the Golden Triangle, to an increasingly large extent in Central and South America, but above all in Afghanistan. And here once again the CIA was active.

During the Afghan war of liberation from Russia, America and other Western powers inevitably supported the various guerrilla armies. Afghanistan is of huge strategic importance, principally as a route for the oil pipes from Central Asia. Control of Afghanistan was eventually won by the Taliban, which adopted a fundamentalist version of Islam and was notorious for its oppression of women. Its campaign was mostly funded by heroin production and it continued to take an official tax of 20 per cent on all heroin produced and exported.[35] It remained the principal source of income of the government. Heroin is largely produced in the fabled vegetable gardens round Kandahar, which once used to supply the court of Kublai Khan. Curiously, the Taliban had strict laws about smoking marijuana: those who had indulged risked the death penalty. Its justification for encouraging heroin production was that heroin is a Christian drug and does not therefore threaten the faithful. At present, Afghanistan produces the vast majority of the world's heroin and has thereby incurred the wrath of the *Times* of London:

> Few governments have ever depended so heavily for their income on the destruction and death of young people as Taliban, the fanatical rulers of Afghanistan. Smuggling opium to Western Europe is now virtually the only source of income for these hypocritical Islamic fundamentalists; the more heroin addicts they recruit, the richer they become.[36]

Europe catches up

Heroin only took a serious hold in Europe in the 1970s. Britain took the lead, and has kept in front ever since. In 1956 there were only fifty-four registered heroin addicts in Britain. Many observers ascribed this small number to the so-called 'British system', whereby addicts were prescribed heroin and therefore were not dependent on dealers. It was argued that this prevented an illegal market establishing itself in the country. As one distinguished British surgeon remarked at the time,

> In regard to the prevention of addiction, the people of this country have received great benefit from the Home Office which has controlled all dangerous and habit-forming drugs for years, and has controlled them well. This success is largely due to the loyal co-operation of the medical profession. I have never met a British doctor who has sold a pennyworth of heroin or any other addictable drug ... there are only fifty-four addicts in this country as compared with America where the numbers run into six figures.[37]

This satisfaction was premature. Heroin began to creep into London life along with new 'bohemian' ideas from America. Many early users acknowledged the influence of Burroughs, Kerouac and other drug-using writers from the Beat scene. Particularly influential was the Scottish writer Alexander Trocchi, who wrote of his experiences as a heroin addict in Paris and New York.[38] The new bohemian users differed from the older addicts, who were mostly doctors, pharmacists and other professionals. The cosy relationship between prescriber and patient had been one between equals. The new addicts actively sought out doctors whom they could pressurise. The new relationship was one of cajoling and reluctant compliance. Burroughs had described the art of finding a 'writing croaker' in his description of life as a junkie.[39] This skill had now crossed the Atlantic, along with jazz and gangster movies.

In a few cases, doctors became enthusiastic prescribers, either for reasons of personal profit or because of a desire to help. The Health Department began to worry about the large amounts of heroin being prescribed, particularly when they discovered that a number of Canadian addicts had arrived in the country in pursuit of an easy source of supply. Their enquiries revealed that only a small number of doctors were involved: 'Not more than 6 doctors have prescribed these very large amounts of dangerous drugs ... a single physician[40] prescribed 6 kg heroin in one year.'[41] In spite of these small numbers, government concerns led to a radical revision of the British system. The Brain report of 1965 led to the establishment of special clinics, which took over the prescribing of heroin under special licence.[41]

Moreover, the clinics themselves became far more circumspect about prescribing heroin. Like the junkies, they too came under the influence of American ideas and, for the most part, shifted over to prescribing methadone, which was seen as a more 'medical' treatment. Since that time, heroin prescription in Britain has remained legal but infrequent.

It has been argued that it was this clampdown on prescription which led to the establishment of a criminal market and hence, paradoxically, to the remorseless expansion of addiction since that time. There was certainly a drug vacuum between the withdrawal of GPs from supply and the establishment of the special clinics. For a time the gap was filled with other phamaceuticals, such as methedrine, Diconal and barbiturates. GPs were still allowed to prescribe methedrine (amphetamine) ampoules. One doctor in particular became notorious for prescribing huge numbers of ampoules, often consulting his patients in coffee bars and on park benches. Amphetamine was more acceptable on the club scene than heroin and some think that it was methedrine 'which provided the link between the needle culture and the kids in the clubs'.[42]

The market had become primed for criminal entrepreneurs. Chinese smoking heroin was first seized in 1967.[43] Since that time, the vast majority of heroin used in Britain has been illicitly manufactured. Supplies originally came from Hong Kong and Turkey; then, after effective police action in those countries, from South-East Asia. Iran took over next, and then later Pakistan. Currently, the vast majority of heroin arrives from Afghanistan via the former Soviet Union and the Balkans. In 1967 there were still only 1,299 registered addicts, although ominously almost a third of these were under 20 years old. The rate of increase was fairly slow during the 1970s, but rapid during the 1980s when a new generation found it acceptable to smoke heroin. Many of these switched later to injecting. In 1980 there were 5,000 known addicts and by the late 1990s 50,000. The total number of users is now very much larger, and still rising by 20 per cent a year.

Tomorrow the world

It is fanciful to blame this huge rise on the abolition of the British system. In effect it is part of a worldwide trend that has scarcely been influenced by government policy and has been as irresistible as the spread of Coca-Cola. There were also rapid rises in heroin use in Germany, Belgium, France, Italy, Sweden and Switzerland, starting during the late 1970s, and in other European countries in the 1980s and 1990s. In Australia it started mostly among creative circles in the late 1960s and then moved out to the wider population in the next decade.[44] Heroin use spread rapidly through Asia in the 1980s, speeded on by new restrictions on opium smoking. By 1990 it had become common in Thailand, Singapore, Malaysia and Pakistan, in spite of savage penalties for possession in many of these countries.[6] A survey at the beginning of the 1990s found drug-injecting in eighty separate countries, mostly of heroin but also amphetamine.[45]

Populations particularly at risk were those near drug-producing regions or situated on trafficking routes. Heroin use was spreading through Russia and the former territories of the Soviet Union, encouraged by a rise in gangsterism and the traffic from Afghanistan. It had penetrated Laos, Myanmar, Nepal, Sri Lanka and Vietnam, and had once again become a problem in China after thirty years of relative abstention following the Maoist revolution. Heroin use in India was most common in Manipur state along the border with Myanmar and along the highway down to Nagaland, which was a major route for trafficking. More recently, it had spread to Madras, following migration from Manipur and Sri Lanka, and the associated importation of heroin from the Golden Triangle. It is now found in all Indian cities.

In Africa, use was mostly confined at that time to Nigeria, Senegal, Tunisia, South Africa, Egypt and Mauritius, but since then has penetrated other countries, with the help of war and the collapse of social order. In the Caribbean heroin use was common only in Puerto Rico, which tended to follow New York cultural patterns. More recently, it has become a problem elsewhere, particularly in Jamaica. Heroin use was rare in South America, which has traditionally favoured home-grown cocaine. Over the last few years the cocaine barons have started diversifying into heroin and heroin addiction is beginning to appear near sites of production and on trafficking routes. There are few countries now which share with pre-war Ethiopia and Newfoundland 'the felicity of having no narcotics problem' – not even (alas!) Ethiopia and Newfoundland.

In countries where heroin use is established, it has started to move out from the marginalised and socially excluded, towards mainstream social groups which have hitherto been deterred by its image of degradation. In Europe and America use is becoming more common among the middle classes. Women increasingly adopt what was mainly a male habit. Membership of certain cultural groups has hitherto provided protection, but these too are beginning to succumb. An example is provided by Muslims living in Britain, who have traditionally shown very low levels of drug use. Some young Muslims have claimed that because it is not explicitly banned in the Koran, heroin is a better drug than alcohol. A more persuasive reason is that given in an interview by a 16-year-old Muslim lad from Blackburn, Lancashire: 'Drugs are everywhere now – it's just society, isn't it.'[46]

We have spoken little about post-war national and international efforts to curb this epidemic. This is because they have been depressingly ineffective. The American Drug Enforcement Agency has been active with all sorts of derring-do, from crop-spraying to military funding, but, as we have seen, it has often had to give way to other American interests frequently represented by the CIA.[47] Reagan's 'War on Drugs' led to increased drug seizures at the borders, but mostly this was bulky marijuana rather than compact cocaine and heroin. By reducing marijuana supplies, it perversely led to an increase in cocaine and heroin. It also turned the United States into one of the largest home producers of marijuana.

There is no evidence that seizures of drugs have reduced the supply of heroin to the streets, except temporarily. In Britain the price of heroin has fallen from £90 a gram in 1986 to £60 in 1996 and £40 now, while the purity has remained the same. In the United States the purity of heroin has risen from 20 per cent in 1981 to 50 per cent in 1998, and this has been associated with a fall in price. This does not suggest the imminent arrival of a heroin drought, in spite of all the efforts of enforcement agencies. Stamping out sources of supply is a bit like squeezing a balloon. The more heroin production is constricted in one area, the faster it expands in another. Pressure on Hong Kong and Turkey led to expansion in the Golden Triangle, pressure on Pakistan to expansion in Afghanistan.

The Criminal Justice System has been no more successful. Some countries have adopted a liberal approach. Examples are Holland and Portugal, where possession of heroin for personal use has been *de facto* decriminalised. Others have been much tougher. China celebrated the 150th anniversary of the Opium Wars with a mass rally in Yunnan during which forty drug offenders were sentenced and executed.[48] The United States has the highest rate of incarceration in the world. In 1995 it is reckoned that nearly a third of the male black population between 15 and 30 years old was behind bars, and that the great majority was imprisoned for drug-related offences.[49] But in spite of all these measures, whether gentle or tough, heroin use has continued to increase in Holland, the United States and China. China is now suffering a devastating epidemic of HIV infection among drug users who live near the 'road of death' that brings heroin from Burma towards Beijing.[50] None of these countries would claim to have the right answer.

United Nations activity against drugs is vested mainly in the International Narcotic Control Board. This organisation has done its best to collect statistics, to monitor production and trade of controlled drugs, and to persuade nations to sign and adhere to treaties and conventions. It continues to be successful with regard to licit pharmaceuticals, but to have little success in curbing the illegal trade. It is hard to miss the tone of polite frustration in the complaints about member countries that are made in its annual reports. For example:

> The Board is concerned that 72 States and territories have not furnished any annual statistics for 1998, thus limiting the monitoring capacity of the Board. Parties to the 1961 Convention that consistently fail to furnish statistical data on narcotic drugs to the Board are reminded of their obligation ... . The Board notes with concern that, in many countries in Africa, seized drugs disappear and known drug traffickers are acquitted frequently or, when on bail, never show up for trial. The Board hopes that the Governments concerned will address the underlying causes of that development.[51]

Nobody seriously expects the named countries to 'address the underlying causes', nor countries such as Mozambique and Sierra Leone to start providing reliable statistics. In countries ravaged by war and natural disaster, there are much more important priorities. Here, indeed, lies the overriding problem. As Cindy Fazey, an expert on international drug policy, has remarked: 'It is no good expecting governments to control the drug trade. They either do not know how to, or do not want to.'[52] Some countries have other priorities that are understandable. Any government in the position of the Taliban could be forgiven for making use of every financial opportunity to repair a war-ravaged country. The health of Western drug addicts must seem unimportant when confronted with mass malnutrition and a non-existent health service. Similarly, American and other Western governments are probably right to place the interests of national security above their desire to stop the drug trade. They are only guilty of hypocrisy in regularly denying that they do so.

Other countries are ruled by corrupt regimes that blatantly enrich themselves through the drug trade. It is no secret that the government of Myanmar is heavily involved in drug trafficking. The Suharto family that ruled in Indonesia also grew rich on trade, which included drugs. It is likely that figures high up in the Thailand government and the Chinese People's Liberation Army are also implicated. In some

South American 'narcocracies', it is hard to separate the rulers from the traffickers. Many African regimes have been heavily involved, most blatantly the regime of ex-President Mobutu in what used to be called Zaire. In effect, the list is endless and in a fractured world is likely to remain that way.

There is no doubt that the supply of heroin will continue to be abundant. Society must find other ways to handle the problem than just hoping it will disappear.

Notes

1   'Prevalence of morphin and cocain habits' (editorial), *Journal of American Medical Association* 60 (1913): 1,363–4.
2   In 1895 police in New York raided a 'finely-fitted opium joint'. The owners were a man and woman who 'were well dressed and indignant at what they termed the outrage of their arrest'. The elegance of the apparatus available gives an idea of the social status of some opium smokers at that time. The police recovered 'three heavily embossed opium pipes – one with copper, one with gold, and one with silver – half a dozen lamps of great beauty, three ivory sticks, a pair of scales for weighing the opium, made of ivory inlaid with gold, four empty cans that had contained prepared opium, about one pound of crude opium, a dozen lichee nutshells full of opium, a jimmy, a pair of iron knuckles, a sweatboard cloth, a roulette cloth and a revolver'. See 'Finely-fitted "Opium Joint"', *New York Times* (18 February 1895, p. 2).
3   Coca-Cola contained cocaine until 1903. The healthy sounding Scotch Oats Essence contained morphine and cannabis. Samuel Hopkins Adams was a leading campaigner against these home medications. On one occasion he wrote off for the St Paul's Association Cure for morphine addiction, pretending he had a twelve-grain-a-day morphine habit. He received a cure which he had analysed. At recommended dosage it would have provided a daily dose of eleven and a third grains of morphine. Nowhere on the packet was it acknowledged that it contained morphine. See S.H. Adams (1906) 'The scavengers', *Collier's Weekly* (September 22) quoted in White, W.L. *Slaying the Dragon: the History of Addiction Treatment and Recovery in America* Bloomington, III: Chestnut Health Systems (1998) page 68.
4   The sale, manufacture and possession of cigarettes (but not pipes or cigars) was illegal at that time in fourteen US states, starting with Washington in 1893. The Anticigarette League was founded in 1899 and led by Lucy Page Gaston. By 1901 it had achieved a membership of 300,000. It seems strange, but perhaps sensible, that it was legal in many states to purchase heroin and cocaine from drugstores, but not to purchase cigarettes. See Cassandra Tate (1989) 'In the 1800s, antismoking was a burning issue', *Smithsonian* 20: 107–17.
5   It was in response to this event that Rudyard Kipling wrote his poem 'Take up the White Man's Burden'. One verse perhaps anticipates the 'war on drugs': 'Take up the White Man's burden and reap his old reward: the

blame of those ye better, the hate of those ye guard.' See Rudyard Kipling (1990) *Complete Poems*, London: Kyle Cathie, pp. 261–2.

6 Nishikawa, M. (1992) 'Drug control policies in some parts of Asia', *Bulletin on Narcotics* 44: 35–49.

7 Ironic, in view of the heavy later involvement of Japan in peddling heroin in China.

8 Musto, D.F. (1999) *The American Disease: Origins of Narcotic Control*, New York: Oxford University Press.

9 'Prevalence of morphin and cocain habits' (1913).

10 Bailey, P. (1916) 'The heroin habit', *New Republic* 6: 314–16.

11 Baker, I. (1998) 'A hundred-year habit', *History Today* 48: 6–8.

12 The war was kinder to tobacco. The anti-tobacco movement was effectively killed when General Pershing, Commander-in-Chief of the American Expeditionary Force, cabled home: 'Tobacco is as indispensable as the daily ration. We must have thousands of tons of it without delay.' See Tate (1989).

13 Latimer, D. and Goldberg, J. (1981) *Flowers in the Blood. The Story of Opium*, New York: Franklin Watts.

14 'ONE MILLION AMERICANS VICTIMS OF DRUG HABIT', *New York Times* (9 November 1924): 1.

15 A different approach was taken in many other countries. For example, in Britain the Rolleston Committee advised in 1926 that maintaining an addict on their drug of addiction was permissible in certain circumstances. This crucial issue will be discussed more fully in Chapter 8.

16 'History of heroin', *Bulletin on Narcotics* 5 (1953): 3–16.

17 Parssinen, T. (1983) *Secret Passions, Secret Remedies*, Manchester: Manchester University Press.

18 The other major firm producing heroin was J.F. Macfarlan's of Edinburgh. With true Scottish canniness, they pulled out of the trade in time. Their later reward was that over a period of many years (from about 1950 to very recently) they were the world's only manufacturers of licit heroin.

19 For example, the only morphine derivative specified was diacetylmorphine. Hence, there was a huge temporary increase in manufacture of benzoyl- and acetylpropionyl-morphine, which are equally addictive. This loophole was closed in 1930. See 'Esters of morphine', *Bulletin on Narcotics* 5 (1953): 36–8.

20 'Esters of morphine' (1953).

21 Seth, R. (1966) *Russell Pasha*, London: William Kimber.

22 Biggam A.G., Arafa, M.A. and Ragab, A.F. (1932) 'Heroin addiction in Egypt and its treatment during the withdrawal period', *Lancet*: 922–7.

23 This system was a legacy of Turkish rule and was only finally abolished in 1937 by the Treaty of Montreux, shortly after Egypt achieved full independence.

24 El Hadka, A. (1965) 'Forty years of the campaign against narcotic drugs in UAR', *Bulletin on Narcotics* 17: 1–13.

25 Dr Muller sold his heroin to a Romanian named Maurice Grunberg, who ran a decorating business. The heroin was smuggled into Egypt in rolls of wallpaper and tins of glue. After being found in possession of 500 kg of heroin, he was eventually tried by the Romanian Consular Court. It was

typical of the Capitulations System that he received a sentence of a month in prison and a fine of £120.

26 Dubbed 'czar' by his critics because of his arrogant manner. It is ironic that the British and American governments have recently used this term as the semi-official title of their drug strategy co-ordinators.

27 Courtwright, D., Joseph, H. and Des Jarlais, D. (1989) *Addicts Who Survived. An Oral History of Narcotic Drug Use, 1923–1965*, Knoxville: University of Tennessee Press.

28 These will be described in more detail in Chapter 8.

29 McCoy, A.W. (1991) *The Politics of Heroin: CIA Complicity in the Global Drug Trade*, New York: Lawrence Hill.

30 Trebach, Arnold (1982) *The Heroin Solution*, New Haven: Yale University Press, pp. 140–1.

31 Lee, Harper (1989) *To Kill a Mockingbird*, London: Mandarin Paperbacks, pp. 110–24.

32 Adams, E.W. (1937) *Drug Addiction*, Oxford: Oxford University Press.

33 Confidential report of the Royal Hong Kong Police Narcotics Bureau (1973) *Heroin Manufacture in Hong Kong* (September).

34 The French Connection became well known after the film starring Gene Hackman as the American detective Popeye Doyle.

35 Rashid, Ahmed (2000) *Taliban – Islam, Oil and the New Great Game in Central Asia*, London: I.B. Tauris.

36 'The Taliban trail' (editorial), *The Times* (7 January 2000): 23.

37 'Symposium on the proposed legislation banning the legal production of heroin in Great Britain', *British Journal of Addiction* 53 (1956): 39–50.

38 Trocchi, A. (1960) *Cain's Book*, London: John Calder. Trocchi grew up in Scotland, but fled as a young man from its 'stale porridge Bible-class nonsense'. He went to Paris, where he contributed to the Olympia Press under various pen-names, including Carmencita de las Lunas. Later he worked on a barge in New York. Considering himself a 'cosmonaut of inner space', Trocchi was associated with influential literary figures – including William Burroughs, who admired Trocchi because his injecting technique was so good that 'he could find veins in a mummy'. He seemed a glamorous figure when he returned to London. He compered the celebrated Beat poetry festival at the Albert Hall in June 1965, attended by Allen Ginsberg who got drunk. See Ted Morgan (1991) *Literary Outlaw*, London: Bodley Head.

39 Lee, William (1953) *Junkie*, New York: Ace Books. William Lee was Burroughs' pen-name.

40 This was Lady Isabel Frankau, an aristocratic psychiatrist with a mission to wean drug users away from the dealers. It was her telephone number that Canadian addicts used to ring as soon as they had arrived at Heathrow Airport.

41 Ministry of Health (1965) *Drug Addiction: the Second Report of the Interdepartmental Committee, 31 July 1964*, London: HMSO.

42 Leech, K. (1981) 'John Petro, the junkies' doctor', *New Society* (11 June).

43 The first use of illicit heroin by English addicts can be traced back to a meeting with Chinese suppliers in a billiard hall in Wardour Street, Soho, in 1967. See H.B. Spear (1982) 'British experience in the management of opiate dependence', in J. Marks and M. Glatt (eds) *The dependence phenomenon*, Ridgewood: Bogden & Sons.

44 Until recently, the heroin trade there has mostly been controlled by motorbike gangs, particularly the Coffin Cheaters of Brisbane. Motorbike gangs also controlled the trade in Sweden, until being displaced over a period of two months in 2000 by ultra-tough Albanian mobsters.

45 Stimson, G. (1993) 'The global diffusion of injecting drug use: implications for the human immunodeficiency virus infection', *Bulletin on Narcotics* 45: 3–17.

46 Bennetto, J. (2000) 'Drug addiction is surging in the Asian community', *The Independent* (10 January): 6.

47 One alarming development has been recent plans for a type of biological warfare. According to the *Sunday Times*,

> The best-kept secret in the war against drugs is a research compound in Tashkent, the capital of Uzbekistan, where Britain and the United States are funding an effort to culture a fungus called *pleospora papaveracea*, which prohibitionists hope to use to devastate the opium poppy fields of Asia's Golden Crescent and Golden Triangle.

See *Sunday Times* (28 June 1998). There are also reports of another fungus, *fusarium oxysporum*, modified by US scientists to target coca crops. These schemes raise huge environmental concerns and have been described by local spokesmen as 'chemical warfare on a defenceless people'. See *The Tablet* (4 November 2000): 1,481. They are also quite useless, because cocaine and heroin could be quickly replaced with synthetic drugs like fentanyl and methamphetamine.

48 Zhao, Q. (1998) 'State Vows No Retreat in Anti-Drugs Battle', *IPS News Reports* (16 August); *see* www.oneworld.org/ips2/aug98/ 03_20_003.html (accessed, 09 January 02).

49 Fernandez, H. (1998) *Heroin*, Hazelden: Hazelden Educational.

50 August, O. (2001) 'China's boom spreads HIV to its heartlands', *The Times* (11 August): 10.

51 International Narcotics Control Board (2000) *Report for 1999*, Vienna: United Nations.

52 Cindy Fazey, personal communication.

4 *The righteous dope fiend*
Heroin careers and lifestyles

> It starts on a certain level, it's deceptive. You think you're enjoying it.
> But by the time it hits you it's too late. You don't have any choice. It
> comes at you harder and faster and keeps coming.
>
> Lou Reed, on the background to the
> Velvet Underground song 'Heroin'[1]

> I attempted to produce a 'drug-habit' in myself. In vain. My wife literally
> nagged me about it: 'Don't go out without your cocaine, sweetheart!' or
> 'Did you remember to take your heroin before lunch, big boy?' I reached
> the stage where one takes a sniff of cocaine every five minutes or so all
> day long; but though I obtained definitely toxic results, I was always able
> to abandon the drug without a pang. These experiments simply
> confirmed the conclusion which I had already adopted, provisionally, on
> theoretical grounds: that busy people, interested in life and in their work,
> simply cannot find the time to keep on with a drug.
>
> Aleister Crowley[2]

The primrose path

A pervasive myth influences our thoughts about heroin, which is all
the more gloomy for not being fully articulated. It owes something to
the Prodigal Son but without the homecoming, or to Red Riding
Hood without the woodcutter's axe. Or perhaps to 'La Belle Dame
sans Merci'.[3] The story line goes something like this: Peddlers come
looking for you, when you are young and innocent or down on your
luck. They press goodies upon you. Once you've tried them, you're a
customer for life. Unable to escape the addiction, you need ever-
increasing amounts to keep yourself straight. You come running to
their lair. Your behaviour becomes degraded. You start injecting, and
quickly contaminate yourself with infections. You lose all sense of
morality. You'd 'steal opium suppositories from your grandma's ass'[4]

or anything else to raise cash for a fix. You lose interest in friends and family – your only thought is 'chasing the bag'.

You become a lost waif. Everyone can tell you are a heroin addict because 'heroin screws you up'.[5] Thin and gaunt, covered in abscesses, unable to keep yourself together, you are hell-bent for an early death, whether from infection or overdose. Even if you become clean through treatment or prison, most likely you will relapse soon after and continue sliding on downwards. For the most part heroin addiction is irreversible. It is a kind of leprosy, which eats out the soul.

> As sure as I'm King Heroin, you will come for a taste.
> Many a shot will be cooked, because now you are hooked.
> Sit tight in the saddle and ride me well
> For the white horse of heroin will take you to hell.[6]

This would be a depressing tale indeed, if it were true.

In fact, only a small minority of heroin users takes this drastic path. Community studies have provided a very different picture, showing that many people can use heroin for a time and then give up without ever requiring treatment. For example, the US National Household Survey on Drug Abuse[7] recently found that just over 3 million people had used heroin at some time in their life, but only 208,000 had used during the last month. In other words 93 per cent of those who had used heroin had either given up or were no longer using dependently. This does not mean it is easy to give it up once you become dependent – far from it – but it is possible to remain healthy both physically and mentally, even if you use heroin every day for most of your life.

Nonetheless, in spite of a century's experience, heroin continues to resurrect ancestral fears of plague and death. In 1926 the New York Commissioner of Correction was understandably anxious, because the drug was relatively new, and he could perhaps be forgiven for gross exaggeration:

> Of all the plagues visited upon our land, drug addiction is by far the most horrible … . All drug addicts are criminals, and there is no limit to their atrocities when deprived of their drug. Heroin changes a misdemeanant into a desperado of the most vicious type. It has been calculated that five ounces of heroin would produce 10,000 addicts in a very few days. Boys between the ages of 12 and 15 years once in the grip of this vice sell the clothes their parents provide for them, to satisfy their cravings … . Can they ever be cured? I have never seen one case of permanent cure that I could trust.[8]

Since that time, studies like those reported above have shown that the Commissioner was wrong, but they have not yet filtered through to the public. Politicians often provide further misinformation. Ignorance leads to irrational hostility: 'It ain't no crime to kill smackies'[9] is one message from the streets. Users of other drugs comfort themselves that they are not as irresponsible as heroin users, as demonstrated by these hypocritical quotations from a survey on attitudes to drugs among ecstasy users in Northern Ireland:

> They [heroin injectors] should be shot – or forced to leave … because they are a drain on the community.
> (Male, aged 27, unemployed, consistently engages in unsafe sex)

> They are totally stupid.
> (Male, aged 26, consumed twenty-five pints of beer and no water during his most recent use of ecstasy)

> It [heroin] is very, very addictive – you have to steal for it, things like that.
> (Male, aged 19, has used ecstasy more than a hundred times; admits stealing from his employer to buy ecstasy)[10]

Heroin undoubtedly causes problems, but they can only be confronted if they are accepted for what they are and compared honestly with those caused by other indulgences. 'Pharmaco-mythology'[11] is no basis for policy.

Mind and matter

What is the real life path of the heroin user? Is there a typical user career or a life history of use? Do heroin users always get worse at the same speed or does use go up and down, with the possibility of spontaneous recovery? Are patterns of heroin use as variable, say, as patterns of chewing-gum use or is the chemical effect so powerful that it overrides any variability that might be expected from culture, taste and personality? The answers to these questions are important, not just for constructing a natural history of the drug. Sensible policy can only be based on knowledge of the patterns of use. Treatments will be most effective if they work alongside common patterns of use and abstinence.

We will show in this chapter that many people use heroin in a controlled fashion, that many others successfully give up the habit and that, for many, a long-term heroin habit is compatible with a healthy and productive life. Others find the addiction to be devastating, but they will form a smaller proportion of the user population if heroin use continues to expand.

After a very brief honeymoon period between about 1898 and 1901, doctors generally accepted that heroin could cause dependence. If you use heroin every day for four weeks, you will usually suffer a physical withdrawal reaction if you stop. Once you are physically addicted, it is uncomfortable to stop using heroin. After short periods of use, the withdrawal is short-lived and characterised mostly by physical symptoms such as diarrhoea and 'bone pains'. After longer use, the withdrawal lasts much longer. There follows a period of months while the brain opiate receptors readapt and the ex-user suffers typically from lack of energy, poor sleep and powerful cravings which often lead to relapse. People feel at times that they are controlled by their chemistry and that they have no choice but to submit to the call of their neurones. They seek the drug again, like the laboratory rats that have been shown to press the bar connected to the heroin pump in preference to food, drink or sex.

Chemistry is depressingly deterministic, but fortunately humans are not controlled by internal chemistry alone. They are also not laboratory rats, even though inhabitants of some drug-rich neighbourhoods may suffer a quality of life not much better than experimental animals. Humans have the capacity to choose. They can choose to avoid dependence or to put up with withdrawal symptoms after they have become dependent. Many observers of drug use are unimpressed by the role of chemical compulsion. John Booth Davies, a leading psychologist, sees 'addiction' as merely a way to explain to our families and ourselves our lack of self-control. He argues that: 'The statement "I cannot stop" is primarily a metaphor.'[12]

Actually, the position even for rats is not quite as bad as it may appear. In one of many similar experiments, rats were forced to drink morphine until they had developed dependence. They were then allowed to choose morphine or water. Half the rats were kept alone in cages, while the rest lived in colonies of fifteen to twenty of both sexes in a place called 'Rat Park'. Rat Park was about 200 times as large as a standard cage. Its walls were painted in different colours and 'the floor was strewn with objects that rats seem to like, such as tin cans'. Rats kept isolated in cages were far more likely to choose morphine than those who were allowed to live in something like their natural environment. The experimenters concluded: 'In the social group, the reinforcement value of morphine may have been diminished by its interference with the rat's natural activity patterns.'[13] A rat with an active social life finds there are many activities it prefers to drinking morphine, even if it has already developed a physical dependence. Even more so than rats, one would expect humans to make use of social networks and occupational involvement to overcome the drive of pharmacology.

How can we decide between the view of addiction as a problem of moral control and that of the pharmacologist who understands it as an unstoppable compulsion? One way is to observe how people use heroin in real life, by means of ethnographic research. If heroin use varies greatly during the course of a user's life, then it is likely that social controls can overcome pharmacology. If, on the other hand, most people use heroin continuously and compulsively, then we must conclude that heroin has a powerful pharmacological effect that over-comes all other impulses.

The Americans led the way with ethnographic studies of heroin use, starting with Robert Park and his colleagues at the University of Chicago in the 1920s. As part of their studies of 'urbanisation', they investigated colourful examples of 'urban underlife'. Subjects included opium smokers, taxi-dancers, hobos and jack-rollers.[14] Later ethnographers took a particular interest in the urban black community, among whom heroin had established itself as favourite drug. They set up their pitch in Harlem shopfronts, on the streets in Wilmington and in the back wards of the Lexington Narcotic Rehabilitation Centre.[15] Researchers such as Ed 'Doc' Preble, Harold Finestone, Chuck Faupel, Alan Sutter and Michael Agar[16] built up a rich picture of heroin lifestyles that remains useful today.

Although this research was continued elsewhere by workers such as Howard Parker and Geoffrey Pearson in North-West England, Angela Burr in London and Jean-Paul Grund in the Netherlands,[17] the great majority of ethnographic studies have focused on poor urban Americans. As will be explained later, different lifestyles bring with them their own patterns of heroin use. Excessive focus on the American underworld may distort the broader picture. Nonetheless, the same underlying patterns have been found elsewhere, indicating that there are some regularities in the interactions between heroin and human personality and society. If the American work is studied with caution, it can still provide useful insights into patterns of heroin use in other cultures. It must be remembered, however, that these studies deal almost entirely with deprived neighbourhoods. As will be explained later, heroin is beginning to appeal to a more privileged clientele, whose pattern of use will probably be very different.

An active life

A core American finding that has been replicated elsewhere is the active nature of heroin addiction. It had been assumed previously that heroin was used as a passive escape from reality. One sociological view (here much simplified) was that there was a large disjunction for many between the 'American dream' and the means available to fulfil the dream. This resulted in *anomie*, experienced as dislocation and cultural emptiness. Out of *anomie* sprang deviance and crime.[18] In poor communities, access to legitimate 'opportunity structures' such as education was often blocked. Inhabitants with enterprise turned to crime and violence to gain status and wealth. Those who were 'too frightened to steal or fight' retreated into drug-using subcultures.[19] Drug users were thus 'double failures'. They were deprived of legitimate resources for achieving success, but they also lacked the personality to obtain them by other means.

Preble turned this 'retreatist' position upside down.[20] He reported that for lower-class heroin users, their drug use was 'anything but an escape from life'. In fact, heroin users were often the most enterprising members of poor communities.

> The brief moment of euphoria after each administration of heroin constitutes a small fraction of their daily lives. The rest of the time they are actively pursuing a career that is exacting, challenging, adventurous and rewarding. The surest way to identify heroin users in a slum neighbourhood is to observe the way people walk. The heroin user walks with a fast purposeful stride as if he is late for an appointment ... . He is, in short, taking care of business.

'Taking care of business' referred to the demanding schedule that was necessary if you used heroin and did not have unlimited resources to purchase it. To finance your use, you had to have developed some 'hustle', which usually meant some kind of illicit skill. This could be shoplifting, pimping or prostitution, dealing, stealing cars or whatever. All these techniques require the development of skills, both of deftness and social interaction. Success in the trade provided the means for conspicuous consumption, which was admired by those who lived around you. Heroin was therefore one of the symbols of success. Crime would be committed to fund the purchase of heroin, but also heroin was a clear indication of successful hustling.

Just like any business, it also provided occupation. The daily routine was structured by the repetitive process of obtaining money, finding drugs and then fixing them. It has long been recognised that lack of daily routine and structured time is one of the dehumanising effects of unemployment.[21] Heroin use and its associated hustles are answers to empty time. The devil finds work for idle hands, but in doing so he increases morale and self-confidence among his followers.

Initiation

Initiation of heroin use is also an active decision. Outbreaks of heroin use are localised, either to particular areas or to friendship networks. It is not advertised on TV or described in the hobby pages of newspapers. There are no advertisements pinned up in the local library. The first users in a friendship group have to seek it out. The rest actively follow their example. Those who use the drug first are usually leaders and fashion-moulders in their particular subcultures.

Finestone[22] described the 'stand-up cat', who was a cool role model for many poor American blacks:

> In contrast with the square, the cat gets by without working. Instead he keeps himself in bread by a set of ingenious variations on begging, borrowing or stealing. The main purpose of life for the cat is to experience 'the kick', any act tabooed by squares that heightens and intensifies the present moment of experience.

The 'kick' often included heroin. It still does so in many neighbourhoods, even though role models have changed.

At first, this type of life seems glamorous. Teenagers take active steps to follow the trend.

> Using heroin in those days was a fad. You wasn't cool unless you used it and, you know, you want to be like everybody else, you want to be like your big brother, gang fightin'. You want to be hip, and you wasn't in the crowd unless you were getting high.[23]

Using drugs, particularly heroin, becomes a rite of initiation into a glamorous world of the 'righteous dope fiend',[24] beyond the usual horizon of impoverished unemployment. Becoming an initiated heroin user requires persistence. Learning how to enjoy heroin may also require persistence.

It is a common myth that dealers give free samples to young people to get them hooked. There is no evidence to support this belief. Drug dealers do not wish to do business with young users, because they are nothing but trouble. They have little money, they are unreliable and they have awkward parents. On top of this, the business attracts particularly severe penal sanctions. Most drug dealers at this level are themselves users, doing a little trading on the side to help finance their habit. Surprisingly, it has been found again and again that most drug users dislike the idea of inducing young users into the practice, and have to be actively persuaded to do so. An example of this attitude is provided by Jack, a young man interviewed in Merseyside in the UK:

> It never happens round here – there is like sort of rules to it. You know what I mean, sort of rules to getting involved in the whole smack scene. You don't sell it to kids. And you don't like even give any to a kid … . People have got … there's still a bit of self-respect involved. It's not completely out of hand. There's sort of, like, rules and dos and don'ts sort of thing.[25]

Even the idea of peer pressure does not stand up to analysis. Usually the first users in a group are the peer leaders, often those with the highest levels of self-esteem. Whether in New York or Merseyside, young drug users are not the innocent victims of evil drug pushers. Researchers now point to peer clusters[26] rather than peer pressure, groups of friends who together seek new experiences.

When heroin first appears in a neighbourhood, it partakes of a deceptive glamour. It takes ten years before heroin produces a significant number of deteriorated users, the 'junkies' and the 'smack-heads'. Broken smack-heads are not appealing figures. It seems likely that their presence acts as a warning to new users. But until they appear, heroin remains attractive. This is illustrated by patterns of use in Manchester, UK, which differ wildly in districts only ten miles apart. In Trafford, for example, in west Manchester, the majority of users are aged 30-plus and there is little recruitment of young users. In Bolton, just ten miles north, there are few older users, but a rapid increase in teenage use.[27] This pattern resembles the arrival of an infective disease, such as influenza. On a local basis, some kind of immunity begins to appear as a result of developing street folklore and disdain for damaged addicts. Probably this disappears with time, as old users disappear, and then the neighbourhood may be ripe for reinfection.

Heroin careers

Because heroin use has been most prevalent in poor urban areas, patterns of use evolve in interaction with conditions on the street. Ten years ago, Chuck Faupel[28] outlined a map of what he called heroin 'careers', based on interviews with users in Wilmington, Delaware. He described a career as 'a series of meaningfully related statuses, roles and activities around which an individual organises some aspect of his or her life'. In this sense, heroin users could be considered to have careers in the same way as stockbrokers or lawyers. This viewpoint allows one to consider issues such as career entry, career mobility and retirement, providing a different perspective from that of a battle against pharmacology. He provided a chart of four common patterns of heroin use, which depended on two key elements: the availability of the drug and the underlying structure of the user's life (see Table 4.1). Structure is a function of the regularity of social networks and patterns of behaviour. According to the presence of these two parameters, four types of use emerged: the occasional user, the stable user, the free-wheeling user and the street junkie. This typology of heroin use remains useful when applied to other cultures, and will be used as a framework for discussion.

Both structure and availability vary during the career of a typical user. Faupel argues that many heroin users have well-structured lives, whether they are involved in conventional or criminal work or both. However, the types of work they do are particularly prone to disruption, for example by police action or criminal competition. This in turn leads to lack of structure, low self-esteem and loss of control.

Heroin use frequently causes dependence and therefore a craving that interferes with a user's life if it is not satisfied. Availability of the drug will therefore also have a profound effect on behaviour. Availability will depend to some extent on local conditions of drought or glut, which are functions beyond the users' control and often depend on distant wars in unfamiliar countries. However, personal action can enhance availability. Income can be increased through work or crime, particularly small-scale 'co-operative' drug dealing. In recent years more people are using heroin who can afford it out of their wages. The price can be lowered, particularly by buying in quantity or moving further up the dealing chain. For women, living with a drug dealer allows access to unlimited cheap heroin. Other users will work in minor dealer roles, such as testing supplies of heroin for strength or acting as a 'runner' delivering

Table 4.1

	High availability	*Low availability*
High structure	Stable user	Occasional user
Low structure	Free-wheeling user	Street junkie

consignments. Again, these strategies are prone to disruption, leading to sudden changes in lifestyle.

Occasional users – their rules and customs

The 'occasional user' by and large has their life structured round conventional jobs and activities. Criminal activity is low, therefore income levels are not sufficient to support a heavy regular habit. Involvement in the culture is not deep enough to provide access to cheap supplies of the drug. This pattern of drug use may be found at the beginning of drug careers and also at the end when people are preparing to 'retire'. However, it has also become clear that for many people this is a stable pattern of drug use.

Many people are able to sustain for years a routine of using once or twice a week or even less. As it does not present itself for treatment, the population is visible only to purposeful enquiry. Its discovery is of huge importance, because it shows ways in which cultural controls can override the dictates of pharmacology. Isidor Chein described this pattern of use more than thirty-five years ago.[29] Since then, it has been confirmed repeatedly by those who have looked for it, for example Norman Zinberg[30] in Boston, J.S. Blackwell[31] in London and, most recently, Dave Shewan *et al.* in Glasgow.[32] There are indications that the same pattern of use is found much more widely. For example, when a new drug service was set up in Bahrain, the doctors discovered to their surprise that the majority of their heroin patients were only occasional users.[33]

Norman Zinberg described this way of use as 'chipping'. He showed that the way users manage to control their use is usually by belonging to a group that has developed its informal drug-using rituals and social sanctions. Most controlled drug users try to mix for the most part with other controlled users. Within the group certain expectations emerge. For example, controlled use is approved and compulsive use condemned. Use is restricted to circumstances where the experience is most likely to be positive. Users help one another to enjoy the drug experience to the maximum. 'Junkie-style' behaviour (for example, leaving cigarette burns on carpets, cheating other users, stealing or spending too much money) leads to exclusion from the group. Users have rules for avoiding harmful effects, for example not mixing the drug with others which also suppress respiration or not using alone in case an overdose occurs.

The most important principle is that users avoid frequent use, in order not to become physically dependent. This also has the effect of maximising the positive effect, because tolerance does not develop. A common practice in this group is to use only three or four times a month, but also to indulge in occasional week-long sprees, for example on holidays. Often users will cut back their use further if they believe they are beginning to develop dependence.

These informal rules are similar in an embryonic form to those that have developed in cultures where opium smoking is indigenous, for example Rajasthan in North-West India.[34] They are also similar to those observed in alcohol cultures. Common maxims are 'Don't drink alone', 'Know your limit' and 'Don't drink and drive'. In British colonial circles there was no drinking before sundown. Many of these alcohol rules are inculcated in childhood or at the age in different cultures when people start drinking. These rules represent generations of folk wisdom. Cultures that are new to alcohol and therefore have not developed this system of rules are particularly prone to alcoholism. Aboriginal cultures in Australia have been devastated by alcohol, as have many of the indigenous peoples of America. Other more experienced cultures can be remarkably successful at preventing alcohol-related damage.[35]

The problem for heroin users is like that which faced Inuits and aborigines. At the start they form a subculture that is quite unexposed to the drug. Social rules have to be developed on the hoof by each local network that starts using the drug. A further difficulty for heroin users is that by and large addicted users control the supply of drugs at street level. It is therefore necessary to have regular contact with uncontrolled use and to resist the pressure to use more chaotically.

There is a strong argument that the reason why heroin use is quite often destructive is because it is illegal. Society is therefore prevented from developing informal but effective rules and rituals and social sanctions, but instead depends on legal sanctions which are patently not so effective. It is nonetheless encouraging that many people only use heroin occasionally, even in these adverse circumstances.

The stable user

The second pattern of use described by Faupel is that of the 'stable user'. He calls this the most productive period of a heroin career. The user is dependent, but can afford it. Sufficient income is available to finance dependent heroin use, but also to cope with other responsibilities such as supporting a family and paying the rent. Usually at this stage ways of reducing the cost of heroin have been discovered, perhaps through contact with dealers, through participation at some level in the dealing network or by getting hold of a medical prescription. Because of the cost of heroin, many stable users are involved in some illicit activity, for example prostitution or shoplifting. However, a growing number of users fund a large proportion of their use from licit sources, such as benefits and wages. Stable use is compatible with work. Many have official or unofficial jobs, supplemented by varying degrees of criminal activity. Some users have high income levels and can afford regular heroin. There has been evidence recently of increased use among the middle classes, particularly in get-rich-quick financial circles.

Doctors, nurses and pharmacists may fall into this group. Their job enables them to get hold of pharmaceutical drugs reasonably easily. If they are not discovered, they can maintain a successful practice indefinitely while remaining dependent. Dr Clive Froggatt was a leading family doctor in the salubrious city of Cheltenham, England, and a favourite of Margaret Thatcher.[36] He was destined for a high position in the Conservative Party, before a forged prescription was discovered that revealed his opiate dependence. For ten years he combined his successful career with heroin addiction, and even confessed to shooting up heroin in the men's room at 10 Downing Street. He is now an enthusiastic addiction doctor.

As explained in an earlier chapter, most heroin addicts in the UK between the wars were medical men. This was not an issue for the authorities. Their main concern was to discourage doctors prescribing for themselves, usually by means of asking them to sign a voluntary 'Undertaking'. This was not always successful. One doctor journeyed down from Glasgow to London for this purpose, but on his return journey made no less than four purchases of morphine, even writing the prescriptions on the back of his copy of the Undertaking. Another doctor acquired a regular supply of heroin by claiming he was conducting research into cancer by means of injecting heroin into strawberries.[37] But however eccentric the means of obtaining their supply of the drug, because they could do so they were able to continue their professional lives without significant problems.

The key element in this phase of an addict's career is that life structure is maintained and an ample supply of heroin has been secured. Informal controls and rituals still play an important role, but of a different nature. It will be described in chapter 5 how social bonding can be enhanced by such practices as cooking up together, front-loading and back-loading, and helping out other users who are withdrawing. Ethical principles are still maintained, even if these may seem slightly dubious to those outside the group: don't use in front of children; only steal from shops; don't cheat other users. Many stable users would not only subscribe to these principles, but also adhere to them more days than not.

The free-wheeling addict

A structured lifestyle can break down under the influence of fortune or misfortune. Sometimes, great wealth showers down – perhaps because of successful crime, victory in a legal compensation case or clever deals on the stockmarket. The free-wheeling addict emerges, now able to indulge in conspicuous consumption. Normal routines are lost and drugs are available in huge quantities. Those born to great wealth may also fall into this group. A recent example was that of Lord Harlech, a hereditary peer and landowner arrested for possession of heroin. His sister had died four years previously of a heroin over-dose.[38]

With too much wealth, many find that their habit spins out of control to the detriment of their health. They become isolated from the restraining effect of their peer group. (Specifically so for Lord Harlech, as he was ousted from the House of Lords.) The free-wheeling lifestyle is not sustainable for long. Some are able to revert to stable use, but others find that their income falls and that they are no longer able to pick up the patterns of regularity that they have lost. Deprived of structure in their life, heavily addicted but with limited access to heroin, they move into Faupel's fourth phase, that of the street junkie.

The street junkie

The most common route into junkiehood is through loss of life structure due to misfortune, for example as a result of loss of employment, breakdown in family relationships or reduced success in crime. Reduced access to heroin is also a factor. Junkies suffer a double whammy. Not only do they have less income to purchase drugs, but also they have reduced access to cheaper, high-grade heroin. As their behaviour becomes more unreliable, they are that much more in danger of being arrested. Stable users avoid their company. To get their drugs, they have to purchase at the lowest level in the dealing chain, where quality and reliability are poor. At this stage, life becomes a real battle to keep straight. Getting the next fix becomes much more important than looking after yourself, sustaining relationships or acting sensibly. They often do things that normally they would despise, whether prostitution or unpleasant and reckless crime. It is only now that they finally fulfil the popular conception of a heroin addict.

Probably this is the popular conception because, as junkies, drug users suddenly become visible. A stable user would not be recognised in the street, whereas a junkie is clearly a junkie. Moreover, they are often up to activities that bring them to people's attention, such as aggressive begging, clumsy shoplifting or selling *The Big Issue*.[39] In particular, they may finally decide that going into treatment is worth the trouble. Medical staff may therefore receive the misleading impression that junkies are typical heroin users, particularly GPs who are confronted with a patient forcibly 'on the blag' for prescription medication. They may not know that several of their other regular patients have an opiate habit, which they have not yet confided to them. Their vision of opiate use coalesces around this one aggressive junkie. Unless they take an interest in treating heroin use, many GPs are hostile to users, which is unfortunately a major barrier to rational treatment.[40]

It should be noted that many junkies go into treatment without the intent to give up drugs. Treatment may be one strategy for organising themselves again, so that they can climb back to the plateau of stable use. Indeed, Faupel's stages should not be seen as a Rake's Progress, with one phase leading remorselessly on to the next until final degradation or miraculous deliverance. Most heroin users report that their careers vary over time, with stable or controlled use being the norm but interspersed with episodes of chaotic consumption and hand-to-mouth penury. Stable use may be achieved with the help of long-term treatment, or with intermittent treatment, or with no treatment at all. Some users continue all their lives, but others decide to 'retire from their drug careers'. When heroin users give up the habit, it is usually because they have eventually reached that decision observing their life in the round, rather than as a result of frenetic treatment from drug clinics or sharp shocks administered by the penal system.

Giving up heroin

Many doctors considered heroin addiction as a lifelong illness. Charlie Winick therefore stirred up considerable controversy when he argued in 1962 that approximately two-thirds of heroin users 'mature out' of the habit and become abstinent.[41] He claimed that most users had an active drug-life of between five and ten years, but there were some who were able to give up after twenty or even forty years' continuous use. Rather than a drug career, he proposed that there was a 'natural history' of drug use. Although his research findings were shown later to be based on faulty premises, many other studies have shown that a substantial number of drug users who attend for treatment later become abstinent.

The argument was complicated when Maddux and Desmond showed that abstinence for three years or more is achieved by a 'substantial minority' of opiate users, particularly the older ones, but reverting to drug use is not unusual even after this length of time.[42] It appears now that many heroin users achieve frequent episodes of abstinence. Generally, users do not stay clean the first time it happens, but instead achieve gradually lengthening periods of abstinence. Retirement from drug use is often a staged process. The length of the last spell of abstinence is the best predictor of the next.

Abstinence can be achieved through the help of a clinic, but self-detoxification is very common. In one study, 200 ex-addicts were interviewed, half with treatment histories and half without.[43] It was discovered that the average length of heroin use was six years in the untreated group and nine years in the treated group. This does not necessarily mean that treatment prolonged addiction, because retro-spective data is always open to question; anyway, the treatment group may also have suffered worse problems. Nonetheless, the two groups were similar on most measures of severity of previous drug use. This study does confirm that many users can pass in and out of a substan-tial heroin career without ever enrolling in treatment.[44]

More impressive still are studies which use general community samples, not just samples of identified heroin users. A study of black males born in St Louis during 1930–34 found that 10 per cent had been addicted to heroin.[45] Of this 10 per cent only 16 per cent reported using heroin during the previous year. Another study looked at a random sample of 2,510 US males born during 1944–54.[46] Six per cent had used heroin and 2 per cent had considered themselves heavy users. Thirteen per cent of these users had sought treatment. Sixty-five per cent of those who had received treatment were currently using heroin, compared to 27 per cent of those who had not received treatment. We have already mentioned the US Household Surveys of Drug Abuse which have consistently shown that less than 10 per cent of those who have tried heroin move on to dependent use.[7]

Longer-term users sometimes give up heroin because they think they have 'hit rock bottom' and have no place to go but upwards. Or they may think that they are about to hit rock bottom. They may have got fed up with the lifestyle or found that it interfered with other things they want to do. They may feel they are too old now for this sort of thing or have developed concerns about their health. They may have family worries; often this focuses particularly on parenting, either when a new baby is due or else when children are old enough to realise what their parents are doing.

In one study, it was found that about two-thirds gave up with the help of a rationally developed plan, while about a quarter gave up as a sudden decision in a 'highly dramatic, emotionally loaded life situation'.[47] William Burroughs has called this the 'naked lunch' experience, 'a frozen moment of truth when everyone sees what is on the end of every fork'.[48] The remainder just drifted out of heroin use without ever remembering making a firm decision. In the days when heroin was less freely available, addicts often gave up because heroin became hard to obtain or was of poor quality. As described in a previous chapter, heroin use almost disappeared completely during World War II in the USA, when imports were drastically reduced.

People also stop because their life changes radically. The best-researched example of this occurred after the Vietnam War. Richard Nixon was confronted with the embarrassing fact that many soldiers in Vietnam had coped with the boredom and anxiety of military life by using heroin. It was unthinkable to load up his troop carriers with uniformed junkies when the nation was expecting the return of heroes. A young psychiatrist named Jerome Jaffe came to the rescue. He was consulted because government officials had been impressed with a treatment programme he was running in Chicago.[49] He decided to employ a recent invention of Avram Goldstein: the ERS urine-screening machine. The plan was that no soldier would be allowed home until their urine samples were consistently clean of heroin and other drugs.

In the event, this simple plan worked with astounding success. Not only did most soldiers quickly become clean, but they also for the most part stayed clean when they returned. Of those who had tested positive for heroin, 75 per cent felt that they had been addicted to heroin. A third used heroin during the year after their return, but only 7 per cent showed signs of dependence. Even among those who had not tested positive, half said they had tried heroin in Vietnam and one-fifth thought they had developed dependence. In this group, only 10 per cent had tried heroin since their return and only 1 per cent showed signs of dependence.[50] There was no longer any need for heroin, because there were no associations at home which reminded them of heroin. Most were able to slot back into their previous identities and find once more the support of their families and friends. This episode proved that not only can heroin addicts become 'normal' people again if circumstances are right, but also that 'normal' people can quickly become heroin addicts if circumstances are wrong.

Class and culture

It can be useful to think in terms of careers and natural histories, but in practice there are as many patterns of heroin use as there are people. The most comprehensive study of treatment outcome was the DARP study in the US.[51] They measured and assessed subjects on any number of personal and social variables, but almost none were shown to have any relationship with length of drug use. The only factors that were shown to be important were age of onset and economic status. If you were poor and had started using drugs when young, you were likely to continue using drugs for longer. Even this apparently common-sense association was a weak one, accounting for less than a quarter of the variance.

However, it does ring an alarm bell about the implications of the studies we have been considering. The American ethnographic literature has been immensely useful in helping us understand how far heroin use is a cultural phenomenon. Unfortunately, it may also give a distorted picture because it focuses almost entirely on poor urban areas.

In the US the law has been used more fiercely against heroin use than in most other countries. As a result, heroin has for the most part been a component of underground culture. Until the last twenty years, heroin use was rare outside the US. There has therefore been little opportunity for a tradition of social use to emerge among people with advantages such as social stability and mainstream occupational prospects. As mentioned earlier, there are signs that this is changing and that heroin is beginning to creep upmarket. We have indicated how patterns of heroin use are influenced beneficially by regular life structures, affordable access to heroin and by the development of supportive rituals and social functions with friendship groups. Middle-class users are likely to have significant advantages in all these areas and, as a result, have greater opportunities to use in a stable or controlled manner. It is significant that half the controlled users in Dave Shewan's study from Glasgow had university degrees.

The American experience in Vietnam provides some idea of how heroin might be used if it was more acceptable to society. In Vietnam, there was little taboo against heroin use. It tended to occur as a social activity in small groups of friends. Because heroin was almost pure, it was smoked and snorted rather than injected. A heroin joint would be passed round, but there was apparently little pressure to smoke it if it was not wanted. Most soldiers stopped using altogether when on leave in Thailand.

The typical Vietnam user would fit many people's idea of the healthy all-round American boy: he is often from a small town in the Midwest or South, is in good physical condition, has used virtually no drugs before joining the Army, and shows no evidence of character disorder.[52]

Heroin filled a function, namely to help pass time as quickly as possible until discharge back home. It is not surprising that so many of these soldiers were able to give up when they did return to the States.

Ann Marlowe is a good example of a new-style American user. In her articles in *Village Voice*, and in her recent book *Heroin A to Z*, she describes her life as a heroin user who also keeps up a high-powered financial job. As a good New Age citizen, she combined heroin with a physical training programme:

> All my junkie friends had been good athletes ... Cassandra used to snort dope immediately before going running (I, more puritanical, did it after as a reward); a friend ran the New York Marathon high ... I played a curious game with myself, balancing heroin against exercise in an effort to get high as often as I wanted without losing my strength and muscle tone.[53]

Peter McDermott can stand as an English example. He is a self-confessed opiate user, a regular contributor to hard-drug user discussion groups on the Internet, a journalist and effective campaigner for better drug services. As he writes,

> I have a number of friends who are addicted to opiate drugs. All have been using opiates for ten years or more. All own their own homes, are married, with children, pay taxes and live more or less like any other good citizens. Some, though not all, receive a legal supply of drugs from the state.[54]

It has been amply documented that long-term dependence on opiates such as morphine, methadone and opium are compatible with healthy, productive lives. Differences between heroin and other opiates are not huge. Heroin's reputation as a destroyer of lives is caused largely by its illegality. As a result, it has nearly always been most available in areas with the largest social problems and among the people least able to deal with it. We have shown that even among this group, controlled and stable use is not only possible, but is probably the norm.

However, the only evidence we have for long-term legal use of heroin comes from those prescribed it long-term in Britain. Many of these have been able to function well and successfully. One of the authors prescribes heroin on a regular basis to a number of people who lead stable productive lives, including a prosperous lawyer, a bookshop owner, a boat-builder and a professional cricketer. These professional heroin users are perhaps the model for future heroin use in the developed world.

Studies from the Third World are still rare. One paper from Nepal described a number of different lifestyles.[55] On the one hand, there was a homeless street child who started heroin at the age of 9 and whose income derived from recycling garbage. Heroin was one of his few pleasures and a means of coping with extreme deprivation. Unfortunately, he died at a young age of an overdose. On the other hand, there was a mountain guide who 'dressed impeccably' and saw himself as part of mainstream society. Although he had used heroin for eight years, he was able to reduce his use radically during his regular six-week trips, during which he was leading tourists up the Himalayas. Between trips he would allow his use to increase again. The culture is very different, but we can still observe the distinction between the street junkie and the stable user.

Conclusion

It is possible to use heroin occasionally or to use it for a short time and then give up. It is possible to be a dependent, regular user, but still to lead a pretty normal life, provided regular supplies of the drug can be assured. It is also possible to give up completely after years of problematic use. Heroin is still a powerful drug of addiction and needs to be treated with caution. It can be very destructive, particularly when taken by young people from chaotic backgrounds, with no qualifications, no emotional support and minimal prospects. For the really poor in the Third World, it provides some comfort and is perhaps an aid to mental survival. The victims of industrialisation in Victorian England used opium in the same way.[56]

Patterns of heroin use depend for the most part on four factors: the availability of the drug; the degree of structure in a user's life; the presence of competing interests and activities; and informal rules and social sanctions in the local subculture. All these factors work together to diminish the likelihood of sensible use in deprived neighbourhoods. If heroin becomes more widely accepted in society, it is clear that there would be many more users. Inevitably, uncontrolled use would increase, but controlled use would increase much faster.

Notes

1 Bockris, Victor (1995) *Lou Reed: the Biography*, London: Vintage Books, p. 71.

2 Crowley, Aleister (1922) 'The great drug delusion', *The English Review* 34: 573 (June). These two quotations are somewhat misleading. Lou Reed, who sang so passionately about heroin, gave up the habit with the help of Narcotics Anonymous at the age of 39. He then joined the Rock Against Drugs movement. Crowley, who believed in the power of free will, was troubled by severe heroin dependence up until the day he died. See Bockris (1995) and Martin Booth (2000) *A Magick Life*, London: Hodder & Stoughton.

3 'I see a lilly on thy brow with anguish moist and fever dew; and on thy cheeks a fading rose fast withereth too ... I saw their starved lips in the gloam with horrid warning gaping wide.' See John Keats (1970) *Poetical Works*, London: Oxford University Press, pp. 350–1. In Keats' case, 'La Belle Dame' probably related to tuberculosis. But it is curious how often the 'lost waif' image appears in medical mythology, whether it is caused by TB, heroin or even masturbation insanity. At the end of the nineteenth century, it was masturbation rather than drugs that threatened adolescents. See E.H. Hare (1962) 'Masturbational Insanity: the History of an Idea', *Journal of Mental Science* 108: 1–25. According to one contemporary authority, onanism was easily detected:

> Sallow skin, lusterless eyes, flabby muscles, loose stools, cold and clammy hands, poor digestion, heart palpitations, hollow chest, headaches, dizziness all mark the young man snared by the vicious habit.

See Sylvanus Stall (1897) *What a Young Boy Ought to Know*, Philadelphia: Vir Publishing, p.113. Today's parents might suspect that a teenager with these symptoms was taking heroin.

4 From the 'degraded confession' competition in William Burroughs' *The Naked Lunch*. This is like the stomach-turning scene in *Trainspotting*, when an addict plunges his arm into a filthy toilet bowl in search of an opium suppository. Heroin-wise authors often indulge in a kind of inverted glamorisation of the issue, as if disgusting the innocent reader increased their street credibility. Perversely, they provide ammunition for campaigners for tougher drug laws. See William Burroughs (1959) *The Naked Lunch*, Paris: Olympia Press; Irvine Welsh (1999) *Trainspotting*, London: Vintage.

5 'Heroin screws you up' was the theme of a melodramatic series of UK health adverts. For many young people, it gave heroin an appealing image.

6 From 'King Heroin', a 'toast' recorded in M. Agar (1971) 'Folklore of the Heroin Addict', *Journal of American Folklore* 84: 175–85. A toast was a kind of American street ballad. Other toasts give a more positive account of heroin, for example *Honky Tonk King*.

7 US Department of Health and Human Services, Substance Abuse and Mental Health Services Adminstration (2000) *The 1999 National Household Survey on Drug Abuse*.

8 Wallis, F.A. (1926) 'The Menace of the Drug Addict', *Current History* 21: 740–3.
9 Graffiti found currently in Lancashire, UK, and elsewhere.
10 McElrath, K. and McEvoy, K. (2001) 'Heroin as evil: ecstasy users' perceptions about heroin', *Drugs: Education, Prevention and Policy* 8: 177–89.
11 This word was coined by Thomas Szasz (1975) *Ceremonial Chemistry*, New York: Anchor Press. He also pointed out in this book that *pharmacon* originally meant 'scapegoat'.
12 Davies, J.B. (1992) *The Myth of Addiction*, Reading: Harwood Academic.
13 Alexander, B.K., Coambs, R.B. and Hadaway, P.F. (1978) 'The effect of housing and gender on morphine self-administration in rats', *Psychopharmacology* 58: 175–9.
14 Lindner, Rolf (1996) *The Reportage of Urban Culture: Robert Park and the Chicago School*, trans. Adrian Morris, Cambridge: Cambridge University Press.
15 How do you set up an ethnographic research centre in Harlem? According to Ed 'Doc' Preble (as reported in Faupel's *Shooting Dope*),

It is like asking how you write a poem, paint a picture or throw a ball. The answer can be very simple or very complex. Until now I've taken the simple course by answering 'there's nothing to it, be yourself, use your common sense. Just don't be a jerk.' And if the person is one, then I say 'Forget it.'

16 Agar, M. (1973) *Ripping and Running*, New York: Seminar Press. The other ethnographers are referenced later.
17 See, for example, H. Parker, K. Bakx and R. Newcombe (1988) *Living with heroin: the impact of a drugs epidemic on an English community*, Milton Keynes: Open University Press; G. Pearson (1987) *The new heroin users*, Oxford: Blackwell; J.-P. Grund (1993) *Drug use as a social ritual: functionality, symbolism and determinants of self-regulation*, Rotterdam: Instituut voor Verslavingsonderzoek; A. Burr (1987) 'Chasing the dragon: heroin, delinquency and crime in the context of South London culture', *British Journal of Criminology* 27: 333–57.
18 Merton, Robert K. (1938) 'Social Structure and Anomie', *American Sociological Review* 3: 672–82.
19 Cloward, R. and Ohlin, L. (1960) *Delinquency and opportunity: a theory of delinquent gangs*, New York: Free Press.
20 Preble, E. (1969) 'Taking care of business – the heroin user's life on the streets', *International Journal of Addictions* 4: 1–24.
21 See, for example, M. Jahoda, P. Lazarsfeld and H. Zeisel (1972) *Marienthal: the sociography of an unemployed community*, Tavistock: London.
22 Finestone, H. (1957) 'Cats, kicks and colour', *Social Problems* 5: 3–13.
23 Quoted in B. Hanson, G. Beschner, J.M. Walters and E. Bovelle (1985) *Life with Heroin. Voices from the Inner City*, Lexington: Lexington Books, p. 78.
24 Sutter, A.G. (1966) 'The world of the righteous dope fiend', *Issues in Criminology* 2: 177–222.

25 Pearson, G., Gilman, M. and McIver, S. (1987) *Young People and Heroin. Report to the Health Education Council*, Aldershot: Gower Publishing, p. 22.

26 See, for example, J. Cohen (1993) 'Achieving a reduction in drug-related harm through education', in N. Heather, A. Wodak, E. Nadelmann and P. O'Hare (eds) *Psychoactive Drugs and Harm Reduction – from Faith to Science*, London: Whurr Publishers, pp. 77–92.

27 Millar, T., Craine, N., Carnwath, T., Donmall, M. (2001) 'The dynamics of heroin use; implications for intervention. *Journal of Epidemiology & Community Health* 55: 930–33.

28 Faupel, C.E. (1991) *Shooting Dope, Career Patterns of Hard Core Drug Users*, Gainsville: University of Florida Press.

29 Chein, I. (1964) *The Road to H*, New York: Basic Books.

30 Zinberg, N. (1974) 'The natural history of "chipping"', *American Journal of Psychiatry* 133: 37–40.

31 Blackwell, J.S. (1983) 'Drifting, controlling and overcoming: opiate users who avoid becoming chronically dependent', *Journal of Drug Issues* 13: 219–36.

32 Shewan, D., Dalgarno, P., Marshall, A. and Lowe, E. (1998) 'Patterns of heroin use among a non-treatment sample in Glasgow, Scotland', *Addiction Research* 6: 215–34.

33 Abdel-Mahgoud, M. and Al-Haddad, M.K. (1996) 'Heroin addiction in Bahrain: 15 years' experience', *Addiction* 91: 1,859–64.

34 Ganguly, K.K., Sharma, H.K. and Krishnamachari, K.A.V.R. (1995) 'An ethnographic account of opium consumers of Rajasthan', *Addiction* 90: 9–12.

35 A celebrated example is the huge difference in alcohol problems in Chicago between Americans of Italian and Irish extraction but similar social status. See George Vaillant (1983) *The Natural History of Alcoholism*, Cambridge: Harvard University Press, pp. 58–62. A good summary of the voluminous literature on this theme is Stanton Peele and Archie Brodsky (1996) *Alcohol and Society. How Culture Influences the Way People Drink*, pamphlet prepared for the Wine Institute, San Francisco (available at http://peele.sas.nl/lib/sociocult.html).

36 Heath Minister Frank Dobson remarked in the UK Parliament:

> Their [Tory] reorganisation of primary care was based on advice from a Tory doctor who was a smackhead, Dr Clive Froggatt … . He told the *Observer* he was taking heroin every day 'shooting up before meetings with Ministers'. He added: 'No-one in Westminster noticed anything wrong' … . He ended up being convicted for fraud [for misusing NHS prescriptions to obtain his supplies of heroin]. Therefore, the Tories were advised on their major reorganisation of the NHS by a junkie and a fraudster. No wonder it is such a organisational mess. No wonder we need a review.

See House of Commons Hansard Debates (25 June 1997): part 37.

37 Spear, Bing (1994) 'The early years of the British system in practice', in Strang, J. and Gossop, M. (eds) *Heroin Addiction and Drug Policy: the British System*, Oxford: Oxford Medical Publications, p. 8.

38 At that time he told the inquest: 'Drunkenness and drug abuse, I think, fall very often to people of high intelligence. They feel frustrated by their own inability to succeed' (*The Times*, 11 November 1999) p. 5.

39 A newspaper sold in the UK by homeless people, under the auspices of a charity that aims to improve their condition. Many *Big Issue* salesmen are heroin addicts.

40 See, for example, A. Davies and P. Huxley (1997) 'Survey of general practitioners' opinions on treatment of opiate users', *British Medical Journal* 7: 1,173–4.

41 Winick, C. (1962) 'Maturing out of addiction', *Bulletin on Narcotics* 14: 1–7.

42 Maddux, J.F. and Desmond, D.P. (1980) 'New light on the maturing out hypothesis in opioid dependence', *Bulletin on Narcotics* 33: 15–24.

43 Waldorf, D. (1983) 'Natural recovery from opiate addiction: some social-psychological processes of untreated recovery', *Journal of Drug Issues* 13: 237–80.

44 Many studies have shown substantial achievement of abstinence in treatment samples. For example, see G.V. Stimson, E. Oppenheimer and A. Thorley (1978) 'Seven year follow-up of heroin addicts: drug use and outcome', *British Medical Journal* 1: 1,190–2. After seven years, 107 patients of a London clinic were contacted. Forty were abstinent, thirty-three for over two years. Abstinence was not replaced by dependence on alcohol or other drugs.

45 Robins, L.N. and Murphy, G.E. (1967) 'Drug use in a normal population of young negro men', *American Journal of Public Health* 57: 1,580–96.

46 O'Donnell, J.A., Voss, H.L., Clayton, R.R., Slatin, G.T. and Room, R.G.W. (1976) *Young Men and Drugs – A Nationwide Survey*, NIDA Research Monograph 5.

47 Parker, H., Bakx, K. and Newcombe, R. (1988) *Living with Heroin*, Milton Keynes: Open University Press, pp. 55–7; Smart, R. (1994) 'Dependence and the correlates of change', in Griffith Edwards and Malcolm Lader (eds) *Addiction: Processes of Change*, London: Oxford University Press, pp. 78–94.

48 Burroughs, William (1993) *The Naked Lunch*, London: Flamingo Press, page 7.

49 See 'Journal interview: Conversation with Avram Goldstein', *Addiction* 92 (1997): 1,241–54. Goldstein was also one of the scientists who discovered endorphins, the body's own opiates which are mimicked by heroin.

50 Robins, L.N., Davis, D.H. and Goodwin, D.W. (1973) 'Drug use by US Army enlisted men in Vietnam: a follow-up on their return home', *American Journal of Epidemiology* 99: 235–49.

51 Joe, G.W. and Simpson, D.D. (1983) 'Social factors relating to the follow-up status of opioid addicts', *Journal of Psychoactive Drugs* 15: 207–17.

52 Zinberg, N.E. (1972) 'Rehabilitation of heroin users in Vietnam', *Contemporary Drug Problems* 1: 263–94.

53 Marlowe, Ann (1999) *How to stop time. Heroin from A to Z*, London: Virago Press, p. 265.

54 McDermott, P. (1992) 'Representations of drug users. Facts, myths and their role in harm reduction strategy', in P.A. O'Hare, R. Newcombe, A. Matthews, E.C. Buning and E. Drucker (eds) *The reduction of drug-related harm*, London: Routledge, pp. 195–201.

55 Jutkowitz, J.M., Spielmann, H., Koehler, U., Lohani, J. and Pande, A. (1997) 'Drug use in Nepal: the view from the street', *Substance Use and Misuse* 32: 987–1,004.
56 Berridge, V. and Edwards, G. (1987) *Opium and the People: opiate use in nineteenth century England*, New Haven: Yale University Press.

5 *How to stop time*

Personal experience of heroin use

The life of the senses is not passive.

David Lenson[1]

The idea that specific drugs have fixed and predictable effects which vary from person to person is extremely widespread but it remains a fallacy. In the particular case of the psychoactive drugs, such effects are the exception rather than the rule.

Michael Gossop[2]

What is it like to take heroin? Can it be described at all in words? Why do people take it again and again? In this chapter we look at the way heroin users perceive their drug. In the final analysis, people take heroin because they want to do so. They may like the way it feels, or maybe they crave for it, or there may be a large gap in their life if they don't take it. They may hope that they will live more effectively thereby, or perhaps that it will help them deal with mental or physical pain. Many users identify with a particular lifestyle and see it as a passport into some type of glamorous social set. The reasons are many and varied, and usually change over the course of a career.

It is also the case that the experience itself changes. Like all mental sensations, it stems from a complex neural pattern, which is formed not just by basic physiology but also by the personality of the user and the circumstances in which the drug is taken. Aspects of the sensation appeal to some, but are disliked by others. If one considers the case of alcohol, theories about its appeal must obviously include both the wine taster who savours fine vintages and the park-bench swigger of 10 per cent cider. The variety of use is almost as extensive in the case of heroin.

But first let us consider what it feels like to take heroin. A good place to start should be an account from two doctors who attempted to addict themselves to heroin over a period of a fortnight in the interests of science. They took the drug in the laboratory, attached to a battery of measuring devices. They were both experts in psychopharmacology. It is likely, therefore, that they would be able to give an objective account of the basic heroin experience, uncluttered by street mythology. Surprisingly, their reaction is not at all positive:

> We've been on heroin a week now, Stuart and I. Seven days of voluntary illness. And how ill we feel ... . The extraordinary thing is that it brings no joy, no pleasure. Weariness above all. At most some hours of disinterest – the world passing by while you just feel untouched. Even after the injection there is no sort of thrill, no mind-expanding nonsense, no orgiastic heights, no Kubla Khan. A feeling of oppressed breathing, a slight flush, a sense of strange unease, almost fear unknown. ... You doze, see a daft scene where someone throws something, jump with a sort of panic, and doze again. Hypnagogic hallucinations they're called. Itching and itching, you scratch and turn. Why should people take this stuff? – not for joy. Only for an hour of sudden shafts of panic and itching? Just for some later escape to apathy, I suppose.[3]

Clearly not much fun! If they had been considering marketing the drug, they probably would have changed their mind and looked for something else. This is not how most people imagine the joys of heroin. But perhaps they were just too objective. Maybe their medical training hindered rather than helped, a bit like a sound mixer who is so busy with his equipment that he cannot enjoy the music. The account of a curious layman would perhaps be more informative. One such 'psychonaut' recently posted this description on his website:

> The best description regarding the cerebral aspect of the experience that I can muster is that of a strong, thick, and gluey feeling, greatly diminishing the analytic aspect of thought. The physical aspect was relaxing, and my entire body felt heavy and dense. Despite that fact, the physical feeling wasn't nearly the ecstasy I had expected. ... After about fifteen minutes, I decided to smoke a bit more. ... I was lapsing in and out of consciousness, if consciousness is what one might call it. ... I couldn't think or contemplate in any normal sense. I also felt nauseous unless I lay, unmoving, flat on my back. ... After a while, I set out for bed and slept well, except for fits of itching, which I am told is a symptom of heroin use. I drifted off to sleep thinking, 'How could that experience be attractive to anyone?'[4]

Once again, a dreary evening in. It begins to appear that heroin must be an acquired taste, like caviar or oysters. Certain physical symptoms are common to both accounts, such as heaviness of the limbs and itching and drowsiness. But it is hard to understand so far how anybody could become addicted to such sensations. If we are to find some justification for the heroin habit, we must look for a connoisseur who can explain to us exactly why he enjoys consuming the drug. One such account comes from the pen of Anthony Lloyd, a war correspondent. In his book he describes just how much he craved emotional relief on the day of his return from covering the brutal war in Chechnya. He referred to this conflict as 'glimpse from the edge of hell'. After a period of abstinence he was very eager to 'chase the dragon' once more:

> I sucked in the smoke greedily, and the cold wash of anaesthesia hit me. It swept over me, a wave that started at the tip of my nose, rushing across my face to my head, running down my neck to my chest, crashing into a warm golden explosion in my stomach, my groin, a blissed sensation beyond the peak of orgasm and relief of nausea, as every muscle in my body relaxed and my head lolled gently onto my shoulder, every sense unwinding, unburdened of the crushing weight of pain I never even knew that I had: the rush, the wave, death, heaven, completion. For hours and hours. The hit. Sensual ultimatum. You can argue over every other aspect of heroin, but you can never dispute the hit. Get it right and you may never look back. Except in regret. As I write about it now, just thinking about it makes my skin crawl, and the saliva jumps into my mouth like one of Pavlov's dogs.[5]

What do we make of these totally different reactions? One could argue that, in Lloyd's case, there is an exaggerated reaction to the horrific scenes he had witnessed in the Caucasus. This is perhaps an unusual example of heroin's ability to relieve psychic pain. But there is much more to his account than psychic analgesia. It is not just heroin's capacity to soothe pain that calls forth the Pavlovian reflex, but the sheer sensual power of the drug. Even if we allow for the heightening of experience that Lloyd's wartime experiences might have brought to his perception of 'the hit', there remains an almost unbridgeable gap between the reports. If we had read the descriptions of symptoms alone, we would have thought the curious laboratory researchers had taken a quite different drug from the war correspondent. How do we account for this divergence?

Howard Becker might provide an answer. He was the sociologist who taught Americans the skills involved in 'getting stoned'. He argued half a century ago that people have to learn how to respond to a drug.[6] Novice users of cannabis do not know what it feels like to be high and do not have the language or concepts to describe what they feel. They may be frightened or repelled by the same sensations that initiates will value highly. They may not even notice any internal changes, because they do not know what they are seeking. If they persist, the example and conversation of other users will in time shape their perception and experience of cannabis. 'Becoming stoned' is therefore better seen as a social and cultural construction than a simple pharmacological response; or at least as a complex interaction between the two domains of experience.[7]

Other researchers have taken up Becker's ideas. In a classic experiment two psychologists gave volunteers injections of adrenaline. This is the substance that the body produces when it prepares for activity. The heart beats faster, airways expand and energy reserves are mobilised for action. Some volunteers were told what physiological effects to expect, whereas others were given no guidance. A third group was injected with a placebo without any information. All were told that they were taking part in an experiment on visual processes and were asked to sit for a time in a waiting room. An actor had been planted in the room, pretending to be another volunteer. He was told to mime various mental states with different cohorts of volunteers, for example irritability or extreme euphoria.

It was found that the actor's behaviour influenced the volunteers' perception of the effect of the drug they had been given. Some became euphoric and some became irritable. This effect was most marked in those who had been given adrenaline but no guidance, less marked in those who had been given placebo and least marked in those who had been told what physiological effects to expect. In the first and third groups the drug administered was the same, but their mental experience was quite different. If they had been told by the researchers to expect a quickened pulse, then they interpreted this as a pharmacological response and did not feel at all excited. Without this guidance they experienced it as a component of an emotional response, and this in turn was shaped by the behaviour of the company around them.

Although the drug was the same in both cases, the mind set of the two groups was different. So too was the setting in which they experienced the physiological response. Set and setting were clearly more important in shaping their perception of the drug's effects than any underlying, strictly pharmacological effect. The difference was even present when placebo was taken.[8]

Timothy Leary and Robert Alpert used this concept of 'drug, set and setting' in their early research on LSD and psilocybin at Harvard in the 1960s. Later, Leary 'tuned in, turned on and dropped out', and followed a career as guru of 'the politics of consciousness'.[9] Nonetheless, his ideas remained influential even after he abandoned academic psychology, and were later developed particularly by Norman Zinberg and Andrew Weil.

In this framework, they viewed the 'drug' component of the response as those parameters that are described in a pharmacology textbook. But they thought that for humans 'set' and 'setting' are generally more important. In Weil's words,

> Set is a person's expectations of what a drug will do to him, considered in the context of his whole personality. Setting is the environment, both physical and social, in which a drug is taken. ... Without them we are unable to explain simply why the drug varies so unpredictably in its psychic effects from person to person and from time to time in the same person.[10]

In fact, all three factors are closely intertwined, but we will consider them separately in our analysis of the heroin experience and of the motivation of those who try it. But we must state first that many people do not believe that this type of analysis is relevant to heroin. They accept that cultural forces may shape perceptions of milder drugs, but they argue that the pharmacology of heroin is so powerful that it must overcome any influence of set and setting. Becker himself took this view:

> Where the effects are varied and ambiguous, as with marijuana and LSD, a great variety of interpretation is possible. Where the effects are clear and unmistakable, as with the opiates, the culture is limited in the possible interpretations it can provide.[11]

We do not agree. We will argue that Becker should have had more confidence in the general application of his theory. As the initial examples indicate, heroin can be experienced in many different ways.

Heroin the drug

It does not make much sense to view the pharmacological effect of one drug as necessarily more powerful or more fixed than that of another.

It all depends on how much is taken, in what manner and at what speed. In moderate amounts cannabis produces subtle internal effects, but if enough is taken delirium invariably ensues. Alcohol can also behave as a very hard drug indeed. In sufficient concentration, it is a non-selective CNS depressant with an action not unlike ether. In less extreme doses the influence of mood, expectations and physical setting can clearly act as modifiers of its mental effects. Everybody knows that the erotic cosiness induced by alcohol at a romantic dinner for two is a very different experience from the aggressive euphoria that prevails at a city pub after a successful football match.

What has become clear is that all drugs produce an extensive and varied range of effects on neurotransmitters, and that these effects do not all work in the same direction. Users can therefore manipulate their neuronal response, partly by the speed with which they take the drug and thereby the speed with which they alter the drug concentration in their brain cells.

The old distinction between stimulant and depressant, between 'upper' and 'downer', is now being questioned. A leading psychologist has suggested that

> these terms might with advantage be removed from the pharmacological lexicon ... . This classification is not applicable to complex behaviours such as selective attention, euphoria, aversion and aggression.[12]

She argues that it is better to think in terms of stimulant and depressive actions of drugs, not of stimulant and depressive drugs. These actions will differ according to the mode and time-course of intake, and the mental faculty under consideration.

Nicotine, for example, can be a stimulant or a depressant, according to the speed and depth at which cigarettes are inhaled.[13] In this way levels of arousal can be elegantly fine-tuned. It is probably this ability to 'normalise' the inner state that makes nicotine so addictive, rather than any special euphoric effect. We also know that alcohol can act as both a stimulant and a depressant.[12] Amphetamine is classified as a stimulant, but it has a definite calming effect in people with the so-called 'hyperactivity syndrome'. Many drug abusers experience a feeling of excited euphoria from injecting large quantities of temazepam, even though it is classified as a tranquilliser.

In our treatment service, heroin users constantly surprise us with the diversity of the reports they provide of their experiences with the drug and their reasons for using it. A psychiatric colleague has reported that since working with drug users he has discarded his traditional psychopharmacology textbooks.[14] Information from the streets too often contradicts knowledge derived from laboratory experiment and detached clinical observation. It is tempting of course to ascribe this to the alleged inability of heroin users to be truthful about anything, even their own experiences. After all, heroin is hardly a placebo. At the right dose surely no one could fail to distinguish its effects?

To some extent, this is true. If one considers narrative accounts of heroin use, certain commonalties emerge that concur with standard pharmacological teaching. These include early nausea and itchiness, a warm feeling in the stomach, and often sedation and drowsiness. Physical and psychic pain is replaced by feelings of competence, optimism, power and detachment. Heroin has the power to make its users feel warm and safe.

But this type of report is typical only of the early period of a heroin career. Long-term users are more likely to stress the feelings of 'normality' that the drug induces. Heroin is traditionally considered as a 'downer'. However, many users take it for other purposes than just to nod off and drop out.

> Many women friends would tell me heroin is great for housework. They'd get high and clean their apartments, do the laundry, everything they'd been putting off. Ondine's favourite dope task was cleaning her enormous fish tank; Sam and Can compulsively repainted their apartment.[15]

This echoes the stories of many of our patients, who report that heroin 'gets them going'. They take their shot to help themselves do the shopping, get the children to school and find their way to work, not just to crash out in the evenings. When they want a kick, they will abstain for a brief period and then enjoy the sudden euphoria associated with a rapid increase in blood level. On weekdays they may be more inclined to use at a regular pace, to take advantage of the 'steady-steady' effect. An unusual example of heroin-supported energy was that of boxer Tony Ayala, former top-ranked junior middleweight. Before he received a sixteen-year sentence for rape, he used to combine his habit with intensive training. 'Normal for me was getting up in the morning, running four, five, six miles, eating breakfast, and then meeting my connection to score heroin.'[16]

Users also take heroin alongside a large number of other drugs. Caffeine, nicotine and alcohol feature regularly in their repertoires, not to mention more exotic illicit substances. The potential for constructive and functional self-tuning is huge, as it is for chaotic lack of control. But many people learn to use their drugs with prudence, allowing for both pleasure and the needs of their daily business. One way to control the effect is to use intermittently. In this way the pleasure is less frequent, but much stronger. This partly accounts for the intense experience described above by Anthony Lloyd after not using for several months.

As a drug, heroin acts in many ways and elicits different responses in different people at different times. To make this point clear, compare these reports from William Burroughs as a young man and Aleister Crowley in old age. Crowley in his retirement was enjoying a quiet life. He was injecting eleven grains of heroin into his armpit every day, but he makes it sound as if he was drinking tea:

> Certainly I want heroin; but anything else would do just as well. It's boredom and Anno Domini. A girl or a game of chess would fill the gap.[17]

The tone of voice is typical of the older addict, though not all of them are up to the girl or even the chess.

Burroughs describes something quite different. What are we to make of his delight in torturing cats when he has injected heroin? This nasty behaviour would be less surprising if he had taken a powerful stimulant, such as crystal methamphetamine.

> When I am on junk, I take pleasure in tormenting and terrorising cats. I hold a cat out of the window or provoke the unfortunate animal into biting or scratching, then slap it across the face with brutal force. I give the cats a bath and hold their bodies underwater.[18]

According to his flatmate, Burroughs also used to tie their paws together before pushing them underwater. Burroughs wrote this paragraph for *Junkie*, but later deleted it in case it shocked his readers, a very unusual reason for this author to alter his work. His behaviour reminds us that a user's response to a drug must be considered 'in the context of his whole personality' and that some personalities are strange indeed.

Many people find heroin helpful for treating medical problems, such as back pain, and continue to take it for this purpose rather than to get high. Their experience of heroin is calming and medicinal rather than euphoric. One of our patients found it excellent for Crohn's Disease and was able to give up steroid treatment when she was prescribed heroin. We presume this was a combined effect of its calming and constipating properties. Opiates are also effective in reducing the symptoms of serious mental illness.[19] For example, patients with schizophrenia report that the voices they hear become less insistent with heroin. Standard medical treatments are more effective in repressing voices, but can also cause stiffness and shaking. There are several sufferers who prefer to use heroin, rather than suffer the unpleasant side effects of prescribed medication.

There are also a large number of users who suffer from traumatic memories of child abuse, of severe accidents or of the horrors of war.[20] Barnardo's, the children's charity, recently ran a dramatic advertising campaign. Posters featured a baby holding a syringe and gripping with its teeth a cord that was wrapped around its arm. In the face of public protest the organisation replaced the image with one of a happier baby, without the syringe but with a caption explaining why the baby was doomed to be a drug addict. But the Advertising Standards Agency later ruled that Barnardo's were justified in using this 'stark image'. It was generally accepted that childhood trauma could lead to heroin abuse. Therefore it was right to take every step to prevent it, even if the public was shocked.[21]

It is true that an unhappy childhood may cause heroin abuse, but another way to view this is that heroin is a very good medicine for intense psychic pain. Frequently, as the drug is reduced, the memories recur with all their former intensity. Clearly it is best for sufferers to come to terms with their memories, for example by means of psychological treatment. But, in the first place, treatment is not always successful and, second, people must be allowed to deal with this type of traumatic issue in their own time. In the meantime, many find heroin a helpful support in continuing with everyday life.

Psychological distress is therefore a reason for using heroin, but it also alters the experience of the drug. The satisfaction lies not in developing a gratuitous euphoria, but in finding relief from symptoms which impair the ability to lead a normal life. The drug does not produce intoxication, but rather a type of normality.

Setting: the role of ritual

Here follows a loving description of one woman's ritual of administering heroin:

I'll score my bag. I'll get home. I'll get my dessert spoon, put away with all my works, and my filters and that, and my citric. I'll get that out and even though I've cleaned it after my last dig, I'll always get hot water, clean it again and wipe a spirit over it, you know, just in case any dust might fall on it, anything like that. And like I'll go upstairs, get a little egg cup, you know, with boiled water, you know, let the kettle cool down, pour a half cup. I have an egg cup of water, go in the bathroom, get all my stuff out, lock myself in there. I put the gear onto the spoon. I'll put half a bag of gear I'll use 50 ml of water, 60 ml of water, you know on your works, put citric acid in, like a sprinkle, a pinch of it in. Then I'll light the spirit, you know the little white spirits what you use, it like numbs your skin a bit doesn't it? I'll warm the heroin up, stir it up a bit, you know, to mix it, and, like, when it's gone like a tea-colour brown I'll know it's ready. Straight away I'll put a little bit of filter in, not a full filter, like a tenth of it, You make sure your pin's on the filter, and not only that, you're not drawing no crap up, no bits of dirt. I'll get it in the works, cool it under the cold water tap, you know, so I'm not actually putting hot fluid into my veins. I'll put it in and I'll draw it out. I'll draw up, get the blood in, make sure it's not too red, the blood, you know. I'll put it in, but I'll do it slowly, know what I mean? I'll put 10 ml in and then I'll draw back again, you know, half a ml, just so I can see the red, and then I'll plunge it back in, and so on and so on ... [22]

We have quoted this report at length because you can't abbreviate a ritual. The whole point is that it should not be hurried, that it evolves in a calm and predictable manner. It also reflects the measured nature of the heroin experience, a calm patch in a turbulent day. In the words of one writer,

> there is an orderliness to it that stands as a counterweight to its reputed flights of fancy. And that orderliness is only emphasised by the chaos that habituation often strews through the worldly life of users.[23]

The user here describes each step obsessively and with relish. All the apparatus, from the egg cup to the filter, are intimately linked with the procedure and each adds to the growing sense of anticipation.

It is like erotic foreplay, slowly preparing the organism so that the act itself can be most pleasurable. During this process the body starts to react. In some users the pulse slows and the blood pressure falls, as if already sampling a foretaste of the heroin. In others the opposite happens, as if protecting the system against the expected changes. In both cases, the ritual itself is a physical experience and can become a focus for addiction. For example, the attraction to the needle can become so strong that occasionally users inject themselves repetitively with tap water in the absence of heroin.[24]

The American soldiers in Vietnam evolved a different form of heroin ritual. It related to a group and revolved round smoking rather than injecting:

> The act of gently rolling the tobacco out of an ordinary cigarette, tamping the fine white powder into the opening, and then replacing a little tobacco to hold the powder in before lighting up the OJ [opium joint] seemed to be followed all over the country even though units in the North and the Highlands had no direct contact with those in the [Mekong] Delta ... . Having observed it many times, I know that it was almost always done in a group and that it formed part of the social experience of heroin use. While one person was performing the ritual, the others sat quietly and watched in anticipation.[25]

This type of ritual encourages easy conversation and cements fellowship (obviously important in a military context). But it also suits many in civilian life:

> Smoking suits me perfectly. It's more healthy and I get more pleasure out of my dope. I take longer over a packet and I still feel good. I am also more sociable. Smoking together is much more sociable than shooting up together, isn't it? You also feel more inclined to give some away.[26]

It is altogether a different sensation from the focused narcissism of the solitary injector.

In Chapter 4 we described how the process of ritual can help control drug use and enable continued non-dependent use, the process of so-called 'chipping'. This was the main focus of Norman Zinberg's book *Drug, Set and Setting*.[27] He argued that 'it is the social setting, through the development of sanctions and rituals, that brings the use of illicit drugs under control'. But he also described how rituals can affect the enjoyment of the drug. At a time when most English addicts were receiving their heroin by prescription, he compared their experiences with those of American users. Because the ritual is abbreviated with prescribed drugs, he judged that their pleasure was reduced.

Some Canadian addicts had the same experience. In the early 1960s, when in Canada policies became more stringent, ninety-one addicts emigrated to England to enrol on heroin maintenance programmes. In the end only twenty-five stayed on in England. Those who returned reported missing the kick of the street experience. Taking prescribed heroin was 'boring'.[28] Some Swiss addicts who were prescribed heroin during recent trials have made the same complaint.[29]

Setting is perhaps the main explanation for the wildly different experiences of the war correspondent and the medical researchers. For Lloyd, the physical setting was a friend's flat. He was immensely relieved to be home from the ruins of Grozny and he was sharing the experience with two other initiates. He tells us that after using they sat back and talked and talked. In contrast, the medical researchers were attached to medical paraphernalia, such as face masks, skin conductance leads and ECG machines. They were lying in separate cubicles. The ambience was clinical and the cultural context a scientific experiment. It is not difficult to see why they ended up giving two such different reports. The role of social and cultural factors in the mediation of drug effects is crucial. To argue this is not to succumb to some form of philosophical idealism. Pharmacology is always important: idealists are equally at risk of respiratory collapse from overdose as materialists.[30] But it is not central.

There is another aspect to ritual, which actually feeds the process of addiction. For many users the ritual involves all the following necessary steps: copping or scoring without being 'ripped off' by dealers or arrested by police; getting back to 'base'; preparing tourniquet, spoon, matches or lighter; the heating of the mixture in the spoon; the dissolving of the powder, with the characteristic smell of cooking heroin; the search for a vein (sometimes ever so protracted); the blossoming of a thin line of blood and its final mushrooming into a red cloud in the barrel of the syringe; then, and only then, the depression of the plunger and the final confirmation that this is good-quality 'gear'. Only then can a user finally relax and enjoy the fruits of their labours.

When one reflects on this ritual and on the many potential obstacles that might prevent its completion, one realises that complete success will only occur occasionally. Often the wind is up but the boat runs aground. Anticipation is thwarted and the user is left with nothing for their pains but frustration.

This pattern of intense satisfaction alternating with failure is what behavioural psychologists call 'intermittent reinforcement'. They have demonstrated experimentally that it is more potent than constant reinforcement when it comes to establishing a habit that is hard to extinguish. In many ways, it is similar to gambling. Intermittent wins make you want to go on playing. If you won every time, you would soon stop betting once you started losing. But if you only win occasionally, a series of losses does not stop you thinking that the next pull of the lever might win the jackpot. As heroin use becomes more regular, the hit becomes harder to obtain. To this difficulty is added the many potential pitfalls in the complex procedure of acquisition and consumption. But the habit remains strong because there is always the possibility that just round the next corner the perfect hit is still waiting ...

Set

Heroin addiction may come at a high cost, but perhaps for that reason it is a glamour item that some people feel they just must have. President Clinton expressed the surprise that most of us feel about this folly:

> For most people in our generation ... we all grew up thinking heroin was the worst thing in the world and there were these horrible images associated with it – strung-out junkies lying on street corners in decidedly unglamorous ways. But we now see in college campuses, in neighborhoods, heroin becoming increasingly the drug of choice. And we know that part of this has to do with the images that are finding their way to our young people. In the press in recent days, we've seen reports that many of our fashion leaders are now admitting ... that images projected in fashion photos in the last few years have made heroin addiction seem glamorous and sexy and cool.[31]

He was speaking after the death by overdose of fashion photographer David Sorrenti, the protagonist of 'heroin chic'. A tribute to his death was hastily inserted in the March 1997 edition of *Detour* magazine, ironically surrounded by an already agreed layout of models posed in imitation of drugged stupor. David's brother Mario photographed the Calvin Klein *Obsession* campaign, which kickstarted heroin chic, but it was David who personified the movement. This was partly due to his own appearance, a kind of adolescent wasted beauty, apparently a result of his suffering from thalassaemia.

The pictures sold clothes to young people longing to be cool, but the concept of heroin art harks back to artist Nan Goldin's very uncool pictures of the plight of her addict friends in the 1970s. Fashion editors liked the general idea, seeing it as a rebellion against 'phoney airbrushed images'. But unfortunately the airbrush was still at work. What was scrubbed out this time was the fact that many underage models were taking heroin and in doing so proselytising the habit to other young people. In the words of a psychiatrist,

> They are communicating that this is not dangerous: an informed or smart user who's got it together will know what to do. They are lowering the threshold for use.[32]

Instead of seeing heroin use as an escape or a 'retreatist' solution, it makes more sense to see it as 'a means of forging an existential identity'.[33] In other words, it is a statement of belonging. It is the way some people tell themselves and others that they are members of a special group. This group could be ultra-cool fashion models, but it could also be wild risk-takers, rebels, doomed Romantic heroes, tortured artists, creative geniuses or streetwise addicts. Heroin use can be seen as having a strong expressive and symbolic aspect, whether it be black jazz musicians erecting a chemical barrier of 'cool' between themselves and a racist and oppressive society or marginalised young people forging identities as '24/7s' in response to economic and social exclusion.

This point becomes clearer when one considers heroin use among the wealthy. Although there are strong links between heroin use and deprivation, it occurs in all social and economic classes. In one sense, heroin is an 'equal opportunity problem'. Not all users are drawn from the ranks of the urban poor. But the wealthy have many choices. Why do they choose heroin? One upper-class ex-junkie explained it like this:

> For those stupid enough, like me, to try heroin in the first place, it exercises an allure because it is seen as somehow chic, as intriguingly nihilistic, as amusingly antisocial and transgressive. And it's so easy. If you want people to see you as cool and cynical, as sophisticated and daring, but you are too lazy or dim to do anything serious about it – like becoming a soldier or training to be an artist – how much simpler just to take heroin. The spurious attraction of heroin as a short cut to coolness is assisted by the fact that the drug reinforces the addict's self-esteem, by paralysing any self-critical faculties that might lurk in the psyche. Thus the painfully anorexic junkie sees herself as fashionably thin; the desperately boring addict sees himself as suavely aloof.[34]

Heroin users take the drug to announce their commitment to a lifestyle, often based on the example of some prominent personality. This intention to live in a particular way interacts with the properties of the drug to form the total experience. This commitment is part of what we have referred to as 'set', that is the mind set with which the drug is taken. There are a number of celebrated social and artistic groups that have revolved around heroin. These include pre-war American jazz players; streetwise 'dope fiends'; the Beat generation of writers; British punks; fashion models and photographers; and heavy rock musicians. In each of these groups the mind set will be different.

It could be argued that common themes emerge from these varied experiences, which point towards some basic property of the drug. Similar words are used to describe the experience of intoxication. 'Hit', 'rush', 'boot', 'bang', 'belt' and 'kick' describe the first impact after injection and are all suggestive of a physical jolt to the system. 'High', 'spaced out', 'coasting' and 'leaping' refer to the floating, detached feeling as the drug takes hold. Later sleepiness takes over, referred to as 'gouching', 'nodding', 'gowing' or 'monging'. These terms may seem to imply a predictable sequence of experience for heroin users in a variety of contexts, but in truth they are not very informative and probably function as terms of convenience covering a wide variety of sensation. The terms are also used indiscriminately to describe the subjective effect of other drugs with quite different pharmacological effects, for example marijuana and cocaine. Language in general is not good for reporting internal experience.

A richer vocabulary has built up round the activity of heroin use, particularly the process of injecting. It is often surprisingly mechanical, drawing its imagery from physical labour. Injecting equipment is referred to as 'the works', 'the spanner', 'the factory', 'the joint', 'the business' or 'the machinery'. Injecting may be 'digging' or 'cranking'. Heroin itself is often called 'gear', while acquiring the funds to buy it is 'taking care of business'. This vocabulary reminds us that for most heroin users, whether artist or drop-out, addiction means hard work and any related cultural activity must be fitted into the short gaps between getting funds, scoring, consuming and recovering.

The word 'cool' deserves further examination, because it is frequently used with relation to heroin and heroin lifestyles. But this common use is deceptive, because 'coolness' has a different range of meanings in different groups of users. Alexander Trocchi gave a literary explanation:

The eyelids droop, the blood is aware of itself, a slow phosphores-
cence in all the fabric of the flesh and nerve and bone; it is that the
organism has a sense of being intact and unbrittle, and above all,
inviolable. For the attitude born of this sense of inviolability some
Americans have used the word 'cool'.[35]

Paradoxically, 'coolness' relates to the inner warmth that heroin brings,
allowing detachment from the outside, a sense that nothing can harm
you and the lack of need for other relationships. It is an apparent
statement of strength concealing a weakness, that you need this chemical protection to survive.

This narcissistic 'coolness' is different from that adopted with pride
by many black Americans. According to Harold Finestone, the
Chicago 'cool cats' were committed to

the values of charm, sharp dress, non-violence, ingratiating
speech, progressive music, manipulative ability and generosity,
which in combination gives their daily life routine an artistic
flavour and makes for a 'cultivated approach to living'.[36]

This is a complex social construct. It is not clear that it has much in
common either with the 'cool look' espoused by the anorexic models
who wafted around the New York fashion studios or the voice of Billie
Holiday 'singing itself into the cool, cool cold of death'.[37] Each group
probably has its own experience of 'cool'.

In fact, what seems really cool in another sense of the word is the
response of the psychiatrists described above, as they took part in their
laboratory experiment. Their tepid response must be related to their
attitudes and expectations. They were aware of certain cultural
constructions, for example that opiates are expected to confer
Coleridgesque visions, but the overwhelming tone of the whole piece is
one of negative expectations. Indeed, elsewhere the author admits that
this is not his first experiment with heroin, and that he had sworn
'never again' after that first occasion.[38] Anglo-Saxon empiricism is the
cultural mind set ('no mind expanding nonsense', 'no orgiastic thrills',
the author notes almost triumphantly).

'Set' is the user's construction of the drug's effects 'in the context of
his whole personality'. Turning to Lloyd's report, we find an experienced heroin user, with a number of long episodes of heroin use
behind him, and well versed in what heroin felt like and what it did for
him. He 'chased' on the occasion cited with two friends (also experienced heroin users). He had, as we emphasised, just returned from a

most brutal conflict. His 'set' was finely tuned to interpret the drug's effects in the way that he did. They were all ready to abandon themselves to enjoyment of the sensation. 'Coolness' is totally absent from this account. He is not describing a lifestyle, but a moment of intense pleasure. It was the 'set' and 'setting' as much as the drug that allowed him to achieve it.

Creativity and heroin

Witness the procession of writers, artists and musicians throughout our heroin century who have had their own (often tragic) love affairs with the drug. In no obvious order we can name figures such as Antonin Artaud, Aleister Crowley, Anna Kavan, Alexander Trocchi, William Burroughs, Jack Kerouac (although alcohol was Kerouac's eventual nemesis), Gregory Corso, Billie Holiday, Chet Baker, Charlie Parker, John Coltrane, Charles Mingus, Miles Davis, Graham Bond, Ginger Baker, Keith Richards, Marianne Faithfull, Janis Joplin, Eric Clapton, Pete Townshend, Jerry Garcia, Lou Reed, Nico, Tim Hardin, Kurt Cobain, Courtney Love, John Cooper-Clarke, Sid Vicious, David Gahan, Boy George, Jean-Michel Basquiat, Michael Hutchence, River Phoenix, David Sorrenti, Robert Downey Jr, Paula Yates and Shaun Ryder. The list could be expanded indefinitely.

Nonetheless, even our incomplete listing covers a large number of major as well as very minor twentieth-century figures whose relationship with heroin (and other drugs) has helped to shape our cultural constructions of the drug, of heroin users generally and of heroin's functions and effects. These constructions have emerged from their works, and in commentaries on their life and art. Reports from direct experience include *Diary of a Drug Fiend* (Crowley), *Junky* (Burroughs), *Cain's Book* (Trocchi), *Lady Sings the Blues* (Holiday's autobiography) and Jim Carroll's *The Basketball Diaries*.

Novels and their associated films include Nelson Algren's *Man with the Golden Arm*, with Frank Sinatra playing the lead role in the film adaptation; *Trainspotting*, based on Irvine Welsh's best-seller; Gus Van Sant's *Drugstore Cowboy* (with William Burroughs in a cameo role) and *My Own Private Idaho* (starring River Phoenix, who later died of a heroin overdose); Quentin Tarantino's *Killing Zoe* and *Pulp Fiction*; Scott Calvert's film adaptation of *The Basketball Diaries*; and David Cronenberg's tribute to Burroughs, the film version of *The Naked Lunch*.

Heroin played a critical role in the history of jazz. It is credited with aiding the development of bebop out of Dixieland via swing. As the musician's drug of choice moved from alcohol (Dixieland) to marijuana (swing) and then to heroin (bebop and cool jazz), so jazz generally moved from 'hot' to 'cool': 'Jazz was born in a whiskey barrel, grew up in marijuana and is about to expire on heroin.'[39] During this latter phase it must have seemed to aspirant jazz saxophonists and trumpeters that heroin use was a rite of passage into musicianship. Shapiro relates the story, popular in jazz circles in the 1940s and 1950s, that if you wanted to put together the best band you had to recruit the musicians in Lexington and Fort Worth, the Federal 'narcotic farms'.[40]

In the field of popular music we find explicit heroin songs such as the Velvet Underground's 'I'm Waiting for the Man' or 'Heroin', as well as the less overt 'Golden Brown' by the Stranglers and Lou Reed's 'Perfect Day'. A recent edition of the UK music magazine *Q* even offered its readers a list of the '5 Best Heroin Albums'. Photography has given us the art of Larry Clark, Nan Goldin and the Sorrenti brothers. In conjunction with official and media discourses, all these works of art (and many others we have not listed) have helped to shape our perception of heroin, whether we be users or just observers.

But does heroin aid creativity? Alethea Hayter considered this question in relation to opium, the mother-drug of heroin.[41] Her conclusion is, tentatively, that it does not do so. She quotes in support the dictum of Thomas de Quincey:

> If a man whose talk is of oxen shall become an opium-eater, the probability is that (if he is not too dull to dream at all) he will dream about oxen.[42]

This is much the same sentiment as that expressed by contemporary musician Chris Starling:

> If you're a twat and you take heroin, you will be a twat who's taken heroin. But if you're a really good guitar player and you take heroin ... you might be late for a rehearsal, but you'll still be a good guitar player. Someone who is not creative can't take a drug to make them creative. But it's not interesting taking heroin. It's just time consuming, and it seems necessary because you'll feel shit if you don't. It's a career.[43]

He also points out another reason that people think heroin is associated with creativity, particularly in musical circles. If you are a good musician with a bad habit, you need heroin to perform normally:

The belief that you had to have a habit that would fell an ox in order to play like Charlie Parker was the classic mistake many of his acolytes made. What they failed or chose to fail to comprehend was that Bird played brilliantly on heroin because he was dependent on it, that was the only time he felt well enough to play normally, i.e. better than anyone else.[44]

But in time heroin often becomes more important than the music. In the words of heroin-using Shaun Ryder of the Happy Mondays and Black Grape: 'The only problem with the rock'n'roll lifestyle is that you have to be in a band.'[45]

English critic John Sutherland has also challenged the idea that great works of literature are created under the influence of drugs. He systematically debunked the various myths of Coleridge, Walter Scott, Wilkie Collins and Jack Kerouac writing great works when intoxicated. He suggests that the myth persists

> because we love the idea of the magical creation, even though common sense tells us that it may be as hard to work under the influence of laudanum or Benzedrine as to drive well under the influence of alcohol.[46]

Indeed, as Burroughs himself has written,

> While the factual memory of an addict may be quick, accurate and extensive, his emotional memory may be scanty and, in the case of heavy addiction, approach effective zero.[47]

Not the best standpoint from which to write a great work of literature.

But there is a sense in which heroin may help creativity. It can demand a commitment to a particular lifestyle, which separates you from normal conventions. The artist can comment on the world from an unusual and invigorating angle. Kerouac's great novel *On the Road*[48] may not have been written under the influence of drugs, but it definitely owes a great deal to the drug lifestyle. Others have argued that experience under heroin can later influence the development of an artist's work:

> Far from constituting a withdrawal from creative life, use of opiates can often potentiate great formal innovations in the arts, as evidenced in the work of Charles Parker, Charlie Mingus and John Coltrane, as much as in the protean versatility of Jean Cocteau and Andy Warhol.[49]

Heroin never created a great artist, but great artists can make use of their heroin experience to create art.

In short, heroin may form an inalienable part of a particular artistic style. Burroughs could not have been Burroughs without heroin. His commitment to drugs was made when he was young and was intimately connected to his desire to be a writer:

> As a young child I wanted to be a writer because writers were rich and famous. They lounged around Singapore and Rangoon smoking opium in a yellow pongee silk suit. They sniffed cocaine in Mayfair and they penetrated forbidden swamps with a faithful native boy and lived in the native quarter of Tangier smoking hashish and languidly caressing a pet gazelle.[50]

A generation later a very different type of artist, pop singer Marianne Faithfull, took up the baton:

> It was in that little town that I read *The Naked Lunch* for the first time. William Burroughs was a cult figure among my friends, we were all children of Burroughs. And I had a blinding flash. It became clear as day to me what I must do. I would become a junkie. Not in that high-life way like Robert – little lines on expensive tables – but in a real life way: a junkie on the streets. This was to be my path.[51]

Stop the world – I want to get off

There are therefore many different heroin experiences and many reasons for taking the drug. But one consistent theme emerges from a wide variety of heroin accounts. This is the ability of heroin to stop the passage of time. Ann Marlowe actually called her recent book about heroin *How to Stop Time*. She writes:

> When I turned to heroin I wanted to halt the flow of time, not so much out of a desire to remain young, but out of a fear of the injuries time might bring … . Distracted by the high you don't even notice that part of the appeal is the cessation of anxiety, especially anxiety about the future … . But that anxiety was put there for a reason: it separates us from the other animals. Living in an eternal present is not good for us, however much we may want it.[52]

The French writer Jean Cocteau describes this best, albeit that he is writing about opium-smoking rather than heroin: maybe he is right that those who most need the drug are those who are most conscious of the unstoppable passage of time.

> There is in man a sort of fixative, that is to say, a sort of absurd feeling stronger than reason which allows him to think that the children who play are a race of dwarfs, instead of being a bunch of people crying 'Get out of there and leave room for me!' Living is a horizontal fall. Without this fixative, any life perfectly conscious of its speed would become intolerable. It enables the condemned man to sleep. I lack this fixative. It is I suppose a diseased gland. Medicine takes this infirmity for an excess of conscience, for an intellectual advantage. Opium gives me this fixative. Without opium, plans, marriages and journeys appear to me as foolish as if someone falling out of a window were to hope to make friends with the occupants of the room before which he passes.[53]

Notes

1 Lenson, David (1995) *On Drugs*, Minneapolis: University of Minnesota Press, p. 55.
2 Gossop, Michael (1993) *Living with Drugs*, Aldershot: Ashgate, p. 15.
3 Oswald, Ian (1969) 'Personal view', *British Medical Journal* (15 February): 438, Vol 1.
4 Douglas, W.D. *What it is to experience heroin: debunking stereotypes*, http://www.ncinternet.net/~zap/12a7b/heroin/heroin_menu.html.
5 Lloyd, Anthony (2000) *My War Gone By, I Miss it So*, London: Random House, p. 263.
6 Becker, H. (1953) 'Becoming a marijuana user', *American Journal of Sociology* 59: 235–42.
7 The response of some cannabis users to Becker's theories was sceptical: 'That guy Becker should change his dealer!' Reported in G. Pearson and J. Twohig (1975) 'Ethnography through the looking-glass: the case of Howard Becker', *Working Papers in Cultural Studies 7/8*, pp. 119–25.
8 Schachter, S. and Singer, J. (1962) 'Cognitive, social and physiological determinants of emotional state', *Psychological Review* 69: 379–99.
9 See Jay Stevens (1993) *Storming Heaven: LSD and the American Dream*, London: Flamingo, *passim*.
10 Weil, Andrew (1973) *The Natural Mind*, London: Cape.
11 Becker, Howard (1967) 'History, culture and subjective experience: an exploration of the social bases of drug-induced experiences', *Journal of Health and Social Behaviour* 8: 163–76.
12 Little, H.J. (2000) 'Alcohol as a stimulant drug', *Addiction* 95, 12: 1,751–4.
13 Ashton, H. and Stepney, R. (1983) *Smoking: Psychology and Pharmacology*, London: Tavistock.
14 Dr Tim Garvey, personal communication.

15 Marlowe, Ann (1999) *How to Stop Time. Heroin from A to Z*, London: Virago Press, p. 73.

16 *Boxing Monthly* (June 1999), p. 4.

17 Symonds, John (1951) *The Great Beast*, London: Ryder & Co (1951) p. 295.

18 Morgan, Ted (1991) *Literary Outlaw*, London: Bodley Head, p. 157.

19 Gold, M.S., Potash, A.C., Sweeney, D., Martin, D. and Extein, I. (1982) 'Antimanic, antidepressant and antipanic effects of opiates: clinical, neuroanatomical and biochemical evidence', *Annals of the New York Academy of Sciences* 398: 140–50.

20 See, for example, T.J. Jarvis, J. Copeland and L. Walton (1998) 'Exploring the nature of the relationship between child sexual abuse and substance use among women', *Addiction* 93: 865–75.

21 'Baby ad justified', *The Guardian* (5 April 2000), p. 12.

22 Account by Manchester drug user, from N. Craine, H. Klee and T. Carnwath, *Attitudes to Hepatitis in Intravenous Drug Users* (research in progress).

23 Lenson (1995).

24 Levine, D.G. (1974) ' "Needle freaks": compulsive self-injection by drug users', *American Journal of Psychiatry* 131: 297–300.

25 Zinberg, N. (1984) *Drug, Set and Setting: the Basis for Controlled Intoxicant Use*, New Haven: Yale University Press.

26 Kools, J.-P. (1992) 'From 0 to 600 centigrade in 2 seconds. Chasing the dragon', *Mainline: Special Edition, 8th Annual Conference on AIDS, Amsterdam* (July) p. 3.

27 Zinberg (1984).

28 Solomon, R. (1980) 'The evolution of non-medical opiate use in Canada II: 1930–1970', *Drug Forum* 6: 1–25.

29 This is partly a result of the steadier blood levels when heroin consumption is regular, but no doubt ritual also plays a part.

30 For further discussion, see Geoffrey Pearson (1992) 'The role of culture in the drug question', in M. Lader, G. Edwards and C. Drummond (eds) *The Nature of Alcohol and Drug Related Problems*, London: Oxford University Press.

31 *Remarks by the President at the US Conference of Mayors* (21 May 1997), Washington: The White House Office of the Press Secretary.

32 Spindler, Amy (1997) 'A Death Tarnishes Fashion's Heroin Look', *New York Times* (20 May), p. 1.

33 Stephens, Richard (1991) *The Street Addict Role: a Theory of Heroin Addiction*, New York: State University of New York Press, p. 120.

34 Thomas, Sean (1999) 'Just another upper class junkie', *The Times* (13 January): 17.

35 Trocchi, Alexander (1998) *Cain's Book*, London: John Calder, p. 11.

36 Finestone, Harold (1957) 'Cats, kicks and color', *Social Problems* 5 (July): 3–13.

37 Plant, Sadie (1999) *Writing on Drugs*, London: Faber & Faber, p. 163.

38 Oswald (1969).

39 Jones, Jill (1996) *Hep-cats, Narcs and Pipe Dreams. A History of America's Romance with Illegal Drugs*, New York: Scribner, p. 135.

40 Shapiro, Harold (1999) *Waiting for the Man: the Story of Drugs and Popular Music*, London: Helter Skelter.

41 Hayter, Alethea (1988) *Opium and the Romantic Imagination*, Wellingborough: Crucible, p. 107.
42 De Quincey, Thomas (1956) *Suspiria de Profundis*, London: Macdonald, quoted in Hayter (1968), p. 107.
43 Chris Starling, quoted in Keith Cameron (2001) 'Watch Out, Needle's About', *Q* (February), p. 60.
44 Shapiro (1999), p. 59.
45 From anonymous article about Shaun Ryder in *Q* (February 2001), p. 71.
46 Sutherland, John (1998) 'Turns unstoned', *Times Literary Supplement* (30 October), p. 30.
47 Burroughs, William (1992) *The Naked Lunch*, London: Paladin, p. 15.
48 Kerouac, Jack (1957) *On the Road*, London: Viking Press.
49 Lenson (1995), p. 100.
50 Burroughs, William (1997) *Literary Autobiography*, quoted in Sadie Plant (1999), *Writing on Drugs*, London: Faber & Faber, p. 131.
51 Faithfull, Marianne (1995) *Faithfull*, London: Penguin, p. 195.
52 Marlowe (1999), pp. 294–5.
53 Cocteau, Jean (1957) *Opium: Diary of a Cure*, trans. M. Crosland and S. Road, New York: Peter Owen.

6 *Ripping and running*
Heroin and crime

I would say this, that users of morphine, while they do commit crimes, they are not usually crimes against the person; they are not usually crimes of violence. The man who uses heroin is a potential murderer, the same as the cocaine user; he loses all consciousness of moral responsibility, also fear of consequences.

Criminologist Dr Brewster, testifying to
US Congressional Committee (1924)[1]

Drug addiction and crime are powerfully associated. Those dependent on hard drugs such as heroin or crack cocaine require huge amounts of income to fund their habit which can result in epidemic crime waves.

Jack Straw, UK Home Secretary[2]

Still less can I take addiction as the excuse for bad behaviour. No one would condone stealing or child abuse on the ground of feeling the effects of flu, and all but the severest dopesickness is no more rigorous than a nasty flu ... . Heroin didn't make me beg, cheat or steal. Had I done these things, heroin would have been no excuse.

Ann Marlowe[3]

Today most people take for granted a strong link between drugs and crime, over and above the inescapable fact that possessing or distributing many psychoactive substances is in itself a contravention of the criminal law. But this link is not nearly as strong as people assume and where there is a link it is not at all clear that one causes the other. Nonetheless, the perceived association between the use of illicit drugs and criminal behaviour has long served as a means of projecting social fears and anxieties, and for mobilising support for the prohibition of drugs and the suppression of minorities who use drugs unfamiliar to the rest of society.

In terms of the link between specific illicit substances and criminality, the association with the longest historical pedigree is the link between opiates and crime. Heroin has served as the paradigm case of a 'criminogenic' drug, to use the ugly term favoured by criminologists. Attempts to link heroin with crime are almost as old as the heroin century itself and were part of the early demonisation of the drug. As we shall explain, there is still a lot of mileage in demonising heroin and its users. That heroin use is a cause of vast amounts of criminality is a keystone of what Alfred Lindesmith once described as 'dope-fiend mythology'[4] and emerged out of prohibitionist and moral reform crusades at the beginnings of the twentieth century.

In an earlier chapter, we noted how the use of heroin in the first decades of the twentieth century spread among young, lower-class males in American cities like New York. As historian David Courtwright has remarked, 'What we think about addiction largely depends on who is addicted.'[5] The growing association of heroin use with urban slum dwellers and members of the *demi-monde*, such as confidence men, gamblers, prostitutes and entertainers, helped transform heroin in the public mind into the drug of criminals. This process was aided crucially by the interpretations placed on this association by policy-makers, reformist crusaders and the US popular press. Part of the legacy of this early association was the Harrison Act of 1914. This pioneering piece of national anti-drugs legislation and its subsequent judicial interpretations together transformed users of heroin into *de facto* criminals.

Although this notion of a link between heroin and crime has become transmuted into a link between crime and illicit drug use generally, and the rhetoric has been secularised, most of the core elements of early twentieth-century US dope-fiend mythology persist as part of conventional wisdom about drugs today. The exception is the disappearance of the early belief that heroin turned men into sex fiends and rapists (which it certainly does not – rather the opposite! – for one of the most reliable effects of heroin is to reduce libido). Otherwise, heroin still plays the central part in the debate about drugs and other crimes, particularly acquisitive crime. The early social and moral meanings constructed around heroin continue to resonate. Let us therefore examine this idea that there is an inevitable link between heroin and crime, and that heroin can be a primary cause of criminal behaviour.

Early discourses on the connection between heroin and crime drew heavily on quasi-medical metaphors. Heroin was depicted as having the pharmacological power to destroy the moral reasoning powers of its users, plunging them into a kind of reverse evolutionary process by which the higher faculties of the brain were first stimulated and then destroyed. The 'primitive' impulses of the 'lower brain' were thereby given a free rein. Paralleling this was a developing medical discourse that stressed the pathological nature of addiction. Addiction was held to resemble a disease because of its chronicity and the fact that its users stood powerless to resist the compulsion to consume ever larger amounts. At the same time psychiatrists formulated a conception of the aetiology of addiction that stressed underlying individual pathology in the form of 'psychopathy'. The merger of these views, moral, medical and psychiatric, gave us a picture of the nature and course of heroin addiction that can best be rendered in the language of a 'lonely hearts' column:

> Susceptible individual ('psychopath') seeks pharmacologically powerful and enslaving substance (heroin), with view to engagement in inevitable downward spiral, ending in crime, prison and death.

Nowadays the language has changed. Those who theorise about the link between heroin and crime are more likely to talk of rational actors faced with economic and pharmacological necessity. Heroin is an expensive drug and dependent users, faced with the cost of maintaining large habits, will resort to 'drug-driven crime' to obtain funds for their drug of choice. However one couches it though, from the standpoint of conventional wisdom, heroin *causes* crime. The relationship is inevitable.

Of course, there is a sense in which the possession of heroin and its manufacture and distribution are causally linked to breaches of the criminal law, since such acts are prohibited by the Misuse of Drugs Act (1971) in Britain and similar legislation in other countries. At this level, the relationship between heroin and crime is inevitable and circular. Drug users in possession of the drug, manufacturers and distributors are all criminals by definition. Distributing heroin may be harmful but arguably no more so than advertising and distributing cigarettes. At any rate, this type of drug offence belongs to that class of crimes that criminologists describe as 'victimless crimes', like certain categories of sexual offence, gambling and violations of liquor-licensing. There may be victims but they are victims who have chosen that role of their own accord. The crimes may offend our moral sensibilities, but generally they do not threaten our property or ability to move safely through the streets.[6]

But what about non-drug crimes, and in particular acquisitive crime? Is the common-sense view that heroin *causes* crime correct here? Before we tackle the complex question of causality, let us look at the enormous research literature that addresses the simpler question of whether there is association between heroin use and crime.

Do heroin use and crime go together?

They do. As soon as one glances at this literature, one is immediately struck by the strength of the association that exists between heroin use and committing crime, 'especially predatory, money making crimes'.[7] Research from around the world clearly demonstrates the link between heroin use, especially dependent heroin use, and acquisitive or income-generating crime. Community surveys and treatment samples of addicts in modern societies regularly demonstrate the involvement of dependent users in crimes such as shoplifting, burglary, drug selling, theft from vehicles, street robbery and prostitution.[8] Criminal justice samples from arrestees, probationers, parolees and prisoners indicate patterns of heavy drug use among those officially labelled as 'criminals'. Similar data comes from many countries, including Britain and the United States.[9] Some heroin users are

> vastly more likely to engage in a wide range of criminal activities than is the population at large, indeed, than almost any segment of the non drug-using criminal population we could locate.[10]

The evidence is complicated by the issue of 'polydrug use' and the problem of how we weigh the contribution of heroin in the context of all the other drugs taken by criminals. Much research shows that pure heroin use is a rare thing in this context. Urine monitoring of arrestees also shows that the majority of drug-using offenders take a vast array of drugs – most commonly heroin, crack cocaine, alcohol, cannabis, benzodiazepines and tobacco. Some research suggests that the more drugs that are used, the greater are the levels of offending. But heroin does play a important part. One clear finding is that heroin amplifies crime where it is part of an offender's drug-using repertoire.[11]

But although heroin users are more likely than others to commit crimes, this is by no means true of all users. Let us take a recent English example, from the UK's government-sponsored National Treatment Outcome Research Study (NTORS). The NTORS cohort of 1,075 dependent heroin users were reported to have been involved in committing over 27,000 acquisitive crimes in the three months prior to entering treatment, with shoplifting being the most common offence. A staggering number of offences, one might think. More surprising though is the fact that over half of this sample reported having committed *no* offences in those three months. Another group within the sample was engaged in property crime, but only on a low level. In fact, it was a small proportion (10 per cent) of the sample who were responsible for the large majority (three-quarters) of the 27,000 offences.[12]

Such findings, and they can be duplicated from any number of empirical studies both in the UK and elsewhere in the world, cast serious doubt on the inevitability of the link between heroin and crime. Whether it is expressed in terms of the older 'enslavement' model or the contemporary 'economic necessity' view, it appears to be untrue.

What this and many other studies show is that addicts support their drug use through a variety of licit and illicit means rather than relying solely on property crime. An increasing number work in the legitimate economy and pay for their drug from their wages. Some are engaged in the informal economy conducting fiddles or working without declaring earnings. Many draw social security benefits and get money from family and friends. A large number work in the lowest reaches of the heroin distribution industry. Links with the distribution network are also an important way of ensuring that they can obtain heroin at an affordable price. For a minority of heroin-using women, prostitution supports their habits (and often the habits of their partners). The most marginalised may sell the *Big Issue* on the street, which is a particularly lucrative way of funding a habit.[13]

It is certainly true that benefit fraud and low-level heroin distribution are crimes. But benefit fraud is widespread among users and non-users in disadvantaged areas. There are also many non-users who are engaged in the distribution of illicit drugs, in particular the huge trade in contraband alcohol and cigarettes. It is estimated that three-quarters of hand-rolled tobacco smoked in the UK is imported illegally.[14] Although fraud and heroin dealing are crimes, it is still a very important observation that only a minority of addicts rely on persistent theft to fund their habits. So the official view of the relationship between heroin use and crime needs some qualification, particularly the view that *all* heroin users are engaged in acquisitive crime.

At this point we take a brief dip into the murky pool of research into the amount and proportion of heroin users' income derived from property crime. 'Guesstimates' of these figures fuel political discourse on the connection between drugs and crime, often producing overgenerous estimates of the amount addicts steal each year to fund their habits and thus inflating the overall contribution of drug-driven crime to national property crime rates.[15] Space precludes even a cursory examination of some of these estimates and the curious accountancy that goes into the production of this kind of data. But to give the reader a flavour, here are some of the figures that have floated around in the UK for the last few years.

Tony Blair, when in opposition, made various claims. Addict crime, he once claimed, made up 70 per cent of the total of property crime 'in some areas'.[16] Later, he (and others) stated that addicts were responsible for 50 per cent of property crime.[17] The most commonly quoted official figure, however, is around a third of the supposed £4 billion annual property crime figure.[18] This figure needs to be set in the context of research carried out by the Institute for the Study of Drug Dependence for the last Conservative government. After considering most of the research evidence with a sceptical eye, they decided that the firmest conclusion that could be reached was this: 'the proportion of a dependent heroin users' income which is derived from acquisitive crime lies in the range 16%–48%'.[19] In other words, theft is responsible for only a minority of money spent on heroin.

The problem here is that these estimates rely on assumptions rather than hard data. Before embarking on calculations, crude estimates are made about parameters such as: the number of addicts in the UK; the average amount of heroin a dependent user consumes daily and its cost; the number of property crimes committed annually; the total value of such crimes; the average illicit earnings of addicts; and even the price at which stolen property is sold. But these are all assumptions. Change the assumptions and you can either minimise or maximise the relative contribution of addict crime to overall crime.

To begin with, we do not know how many addicts there are in the UK. It could be 100,000, 200,000 or even more. We simply have no reliable data. Assumptions about the daily average amount of heroin that a user consumes often make the mistake of treating demand for heroin as inelastic. That is, they assume users need a physiologically fixed quantity of heroin daily. But, as studies show, heroin users 'cut their coats according to their cloth'.[20] The amount of heroin they buy will vary according to the circumstances in which they find themselves. An obvious example is that most of those serving a short prison sentence will use little (if at all) while in prison, even though heroin is much more available there than it used to be. But even outside prison, users will move in and out of heavy use over days, months or years.

A further problem is that we do not know how many dependent heroin users commit crime. Moreover, we do not really know how many crimes are committed in the UK every year. We know what the crime statistics tell us about offences reported to the police annually, but not how many crimes are actually committed in a given year. Nor does anyone know accurately the total value of property crime in the UK.

Then there is the problem of estimating the average earnings of addicts from crime. Different samples give us different pictures. Stolen property is estimated to sell at one-third of its retail value. But addicts are not the kind of people who are willing to hold on to stolen items until they can get the right price. Through fear of being apprehended, they do not wish to walk around too long carrying TV sets or videos. Their need for heroin may be urgent and those buying their goods will be aware of their need. For all these reasons, they often sell stolen goods for a fraction of their value. The price of heroin has also fallen, as have the retail prices of many electrical goods such as videos. Given these difficulties, it is an act of faith to put great store in official estimates of the size of drug-driven crime.

What causes what?

There is no doubt that there is a strong statistical correlation between heroin use and crime. As every student of statistics knows, this does not prove that one causes the other or that the use of heroin inevitably leads to crime. In this regard it is instructive to trace the link between heroin and crime historically in the UK. When official reports and the research literature on this question are examined, one finds an impressive consensus: from 1926 (when the question was first officially examined) to 1980, heroin use was not linked to crime.[21] Most heroin users were respectable members of the middle classes. A sizeable number were doctors and pharmacists.

The Rolleston Committee found that most users in 1926 came from 'occupations that entail much nervous and mental strain'. Criminal activity was unlikely because 'addiction due to mere curiosity or search for pleasurable sensations' was rare. And anyway potential users 'are usually lacking in the determination and ingenuity necessary for overcoming the obstacles which the law now places in their way'.[22] Unlike Americans, the British did not associate heroin with crime because addicts were a very different kind of person. When in 1957 a British specialist reviewed Arthur Lindesmith's classic American study on *Opiate addiction*, he first had to remind his readers that Americans connect heroin with crime:

It is perhaps difficult for us in Britain to appreciate how deeply engrained into the minds of many people in the United States is the concept that drug addicts are, ipso facto, criminals and that so-called 'psychologically normal' individuals do not become addicts.[23]

Researchers first find a strong association between dependent heroin use and property crime at the beginning of the 1980s, when South-West Asian 'brown' smokable heroin arrived in the council estates and inner-city areas of some of our most disadvantaged regions.[24] It is no coincidence that this transformation occurred at the same time as these areas were experiencing the long-term effects of deindustrialisation. In other words, heroin became linked to property crime in the UK only when the addict population largely comprised the economically and socially excluded. Exactly the same process occurred in the United States fifty years earlier, when heroin became the drug of the deracinated generation of blacks who had left the country searching for work in the expanding cities. Heroin had been taken up in both cases by that portion of the general population which typically gives us the majority of our property offenders, namely young, unemployed, disadvantaged males.

An alternative to the view that heroin causes crime is that heroin use is a property of 'criminally inclined' populations. This is based on research demonstrating that in this population heroin use usually follows rather than precedes early deviance and delinquency. From this standpoint an opposite view of the association between heroin and crime has emerged, namely that it is criminality that causes heroin use, not heroin use that causes crime! These two viewpoints have come to dominate a long-running (and sometimes long-winded) academic debate in criminological circles.

In our view, the debate about the sequential ordering of crime and heroin use is an irrelevancy. To begin with, heroin users are a heterogeneous population, behaviourally if not socially. They are not all of one piece. Some commit no property crime at all; another group commits some offences; while a numerically small group commits a high volume of crime, much of it of a very serious nature. Moreover, heroin use varies markedly over time and place. One piece of research may show that heroin use precedes crime, while another has the relationship reversed. This may be because different addicts are considered at different times and in different places.

This cautionary note may seem obvious, but there has been a consistent tendency to lump together research data about heroin users from wildly different sources. For example, in 1996 UK Shadow Home Secretary Jack Straw used findings from a US study of Chicano, Mexican and white addicts to support his arguments about the proportion of income English addicts derive from crime.[25] The problem lies in the way in which the results from samples are generalised to the whole population. This problem is compounded when research findings from one society and culture are generalised to another.

Moreover, this debate leaves out the question of what underlies a lifestyle involving both drugs and crime. We take the 'career' perspective on this issue. Using heroin in a dependent fashion and engaging in crime are themselves linked to another set of variables which help to shape drugs and crime careers. For this criminal population 'shooting dope' and engaging in endless opportunistic petty crime have a survival function in their life on the margins of industrialised societies. As Grapendaal and colleagues argue in their study of Dutch users,

> hard drug users should not be regarded as the mindless victims of some white or brown powder, neither are they the mindless victims of their environment and social circumstances. They are extremely active, they make choices, and sometimes they do the unexpected. A life with drugs, of which crime is often an integral part, allows them to shape and make sense of their lives in a radical way.[26]

They use drugs and engage in crime because it is one solution to the economic and social exclusion they experience. In a consumer society the game goes to those who get dealt the best hands. In the words of Zygmunt Bauman, 'If winning is the sole object of the game, those who got a poor hand are tempted to try whatever other resources they can muster.'[27]

Using heroin, the 'hardest' drug of all, is not simply a way of deadening the effects of poverty and exclusion. Being seen as a successful 'grafter' or a '24/7' man (at it twenty-four hours a day, seven days a week) is not just a means of compensating oneself financially for relative deprivation. Drugs and crime are sources of identity, especially masculine identity, in a world in which deriving identity from paid work is an unlikely option for a significant portion of working-class males. Nearly fifty years of US research and twenty years of UK research confirm that heavy drugs and crime careers are embedded in the most disadvantaged communities. This has led a number of researchers to propose a rather different way of thinking about the relationship between heroin use and criminality, namely that both heavy drug use and crime are the result of the same variables. Not only are they concentrated (but not exclusively so) in certain social groups, but they are also concentrated in certain housing areas. The clustering of drug use, crime, unemployment and deprivation in particular geographical areas has been irrefutably established, both by American research (in Chicago in the 1930s, New York in the 1950s and Baltimore in the 1980s) and more recent British research (in Nottingham, Liverpool and surrounding areas, and South-East London).

Using this perspective we can escape the mechanistic debate as to whether 'drugs cause crime' or 'crime causes drugs'. We can see the link between these two behaviours in a more dynamic and meaningful way. The 'anomalies' of non-criminal addicts and non-addict criminals are no longer a puzzle. Addiction and crime are both choices and can be made separately, together or not at all. But one does not inevitably lead to the other.

First we must add some caveats. We are not attempting to minimise the contribution that dependent drug use, drug-related crime and the presence of open drug markets make to deepen the problems of disadvantaged areas. The relationship is two-way, drugs and crime are both causes and consequences of disadvantage.[28, 29] These areas also contain a disproportionate number of victims of crime. Nor are we seeking to exculpate heroin-using offenders by blaming environmental factors. As we have said, a heroin/crime career is a choice, albeit one made from a limited menu.

We believe that the adoption of such a career is related specifically to two sets of factors. The first is the increasing social exclusion of certain groups that has accompanied deindustrialisation, the decline of the welfare state and the rise of the consumer-based market economy. This we have already discussed. Second, we believe our drug laws and our response to drug-related crime may actually worsen the situation.

We are not here discussing the question of whether heroin-related crime would disappear with the ending of prohibition. We are simply warning against a rigorous application of the law and against the fond hope of many politicians that gradually tightening the penalties will somehow get rid of the problem. The United States already applies severe penalties for drug crimes. For many years the UK has taken a more relaxed approach and has tended to view drug misuse as being more a medical than a criminal problem. All this is changing now: British policy is beginning to follow the American model. We even appointed our own drug czar! UK drug policies have grown steadily more punitive over the last decade or so. There is no mistaking the sound of the penal ratchet being tightened.

Tolerance approaching zero

Gerry Stimson is an eminent researcher with some thirty years' experience of drug problems and controls, and also one of the architects of the UK 'harm reduction' policy. He has argued that the last few years have seen a reorientation of drug policies away from health and towards criminal justice concerns. He sees this reorientation as fundamentally flawed and dangerous. It represents an attempt to recast drugs as constituting a major portion of the problem of crime in our society. Because it is based on flawed logic, it will not reduce crime. But it may well undermine both the real success that the UK has already achieved in preventing the spread of HIV infection and the new initiative that is required now to stop the spread of hepatitis. It may also drive occasional miscreants into serious crime. He argues that 'we risk losing a humane vision of how to respond to drug problems, and our respect for human rights'.[30]

New measures that are being introduced include drug workers being placed in police custody suites to identify drug problems and to refer users on to treatment; mandatory drug testing in the prison system; mandatory testing of arrestees for Class A drugs; Drug Treatment and Testing Orders, soon to be followed by Drug Abstinence Orders; the potential to withdraw social security benefits from those who fail to comply with the conditions of community sentences; the presumption of imprisonment for any offender who fails to make two appointments with their supervising officer without good reason; and a minimum seven-year sentence of imprisonment for a third conviction for Class A trafficking. Much of this is based on the idea of linking the criminal justice system with the treatment system, under the slogan 'Coerced Treatment Works'. Incidentally, a drug that is not included in these measures is alcohol, even though its association with property crime is just as strong as heroin and its association with violent crime much more so.

It is not necessary to go into detail about these measures, but just to note their likely effect. The people they will probably hit hardest are heroin users who are involved in minor criminality, probably no different from non-heroin-using peers in the same neighbourhood. Once tested positive, they will be subject to a coercive regime that their lifestyle makes them ill-adapted to follow. Non-compliance will lead to loss of benefit and imprisonment. All this may well lead to a breakdown of family life, loss of means of support and the descent into 'junkiehood' described in Chapter 4. Somebody who was not previously much of a nuisance to society will then become a serious criminal or a long-term prisoner. Moreover, the tightening dragnet will also catch more respectable citizens who are occasional or recreational users of drugs, with similar knock-on effects on their careers and family lives.

It should be noted that Class A drug trafficking does not imply that you drive a Mercedes and wear dark glasses. You can be charged with trafficking if you are in possession of what is judged to be more heroin than is needed for personal use.[31] You can easily be found with this much if you are an organised kind of person and buy wholesale, even if you are just buying for yourself and your partner. And buying for your partner is itself trafficking. Moreover, most dealing occurs at a very low level, with people passing heroin back and forth almost like smokers lending each other cigarettes. The person who won't go to prison for seven years under the new measures is Mr Big. He will be relaxing in his villa in Marbella. It won't be Mr Moderately Big or even Mr Slightly Big. They are too well organised to walk round the streets with lots of heroin on their person. In nine cases out of ten it will be Mr Small.

In Italy, Portugal, Spain and some German states, possession of heroin for personal use has been decriminalised. But the UK has changed direction and is now heading towards what increasingly appears to be not a 'war on drugs' but a 'war on drug users'. Yet we have no good reasons whatsoever for thinking that punishing heroin users will change their habits. Those who doubt this should consult the modern history of Iran. In 1979 Ayatollah Khalkhali took over control of the drug problem. According to the *Washington Post*, his method was to hold brief trials of alleged traffickers and invariably find them guilty. Often shouting 'I shall exterminate you vermin', he then ordered summary executions which were carried out within minutes. In one seven-week period he sent to execution 176 people for offences related to opium and heroin. But even these heroic measures failed to control opiate use and trade. Interviewed by the world press on 8 July 1980, while licking an ice-cream, he explained the practical limitations to his policy: 'If we wanted to kill everybody who had five grams of heroin, we'd have to kill five thousand people and that would be difficult.'[32]

This sort of figure has not discouraged the American lawmakers. There are almost 2 million people behind bars, more than the total combined population of Wyoming, Alaska and North Dakota.[33] The prison system should perhaps lay claim to a fifty-second star on the flag. Eighty per cent of prisoners are estimated to have serious drug or drink problems. The UK itself already has the largest prison population in Europe. The new measures will increase it further, but sadly not at the benefit of reduced crime. It is right to punish crime and to punish drug users who are criminals. But we do think it counterproductive and unjust to treat minor criminals who like heroin in quite a different way from those who use alcohol, nicotine or even cannabis as their drug of choice.

The long-standing perception that heroin is a major cause of crime has had a very negative effect on the disadvantaged communities in which heroin is most commonly used. Many members of these communities are already marginalised from society as a result of poverty, poor education and lack of skills. Many have had traumatic childhoods and many belong to ethnic minorities. Those who use heroin are likely to have contracted Hepatitis C infection already, since it is currently present in about 70 per cent of injecting drug users. A crusade against heroin users will increase this marginalisation. We need to be aware that the more we pursue punitive policies towards heroin and other drug users, the more we are at risk of amplifying deviant behaviour.

Controlling the excluded

We have argued that current orthodoxy exaggerates the magnitude of drug-driven crime and demonises all heroin users as prolific criminals in the process. The current thrust of policy towards ever more punitive measures can only exacerbate, rather than mitigate, the problem. If we are correct in our views, then the question arises: Why do so many modern societies conduct such 'wars'? Is the judgement of historians like Musto and Courtwright correct that the function of drug controls in the past has often been the control of feared minorities?

One answer comes from critics of modernity and its aspects, such as Zygmunt Bauman and the Norwegian criminologist Nils Christie. What they have separately argued is that in consumer societies the fight against crime (and drugs) is essentially fought against the 'new poor'. This is the class of flawed consumers who are excluded from the 'game' of consumerism. In such societies, they say, the prison system deputises for the shrinking welfare system and the poor become defined as the criminal classes. What happens to them is a reminder, to all of us who are minor players at the table, of what happens if we lose interest or competence as players. Wars on drugs are one way of controlling the excluded. As Christie puts it,

> the war on drugs creates alternative possibilities for control of the dangerous population. The war on drugs is at the same time a war

on attributes *correlated* with drug use; being young, being from the inner city, exhibiting lifestyles unacceptable to the middle class. By fighting drugs … a large proportion of the dangerous classes will be in the catch.[34]

In such a situation, it is necessary that drug use should be linked to crime and the larger the proportion of crime that can be linked, so much the better. It is not necessary to ameliorate the lives of heroin and other serious drug users in order to limit the damage caused. On the contrary, they need to be reminded of their social responsibilities, via mandatory urine testing for heroin and cocaine, coerced treatment, coerced abstinence or the prison system. Urine testing, Christie observes, is the technology *par excellence* in controlling the new poor. With urine testing of people on probation or on licence or on parole, the possibility exists of putting them into prison not for their original crime but for aspects of their lifestyle.

This is far from being a crude conspiracy theory. There are excellent and compelling reasons for seeking to regulate the availability of drugs such as heroin and cocaine. The motives of the vast majority of those engaged in drugs control are unimpeachable. In Christie's words, 'Consequences are not causes'. Reasons and motives may be of the highest order, yet what is done in their name may still be overwhelmingly negative. Nevertheless, the more one studies this problem, the more one is forced towards the idea that wars on drugs have other functions, particularly at a time when crime is actually on the decrease.

How else is one to explain steadily rising prison populations (dramatically rising in the case of the United States), often fuelled by drug war casualties; the adoption of measures which restrict civil liberty; and an accompanying generalised political intolerance towards marginalised groups such as the homeless, disadvantaged young people, people with certain forms of mental illness and drug users? According to Diana Gordon, an American criminologist and policy analyst, 'getting tough' on crime and drugs signifies the return of the old nineteenth-century concept of the 'dangerous classes'.[35]

This designation is neither historically fixed nor a reflection of any actual danger posed by such groups and their behaviours. Such classes appear, or rather are designated, she suggests, in times of social and economic upheaval and change. Labelling sections of the young as belonging to 'yob culture'; designating the excluded as 'the underclass' and drug users as criminals; imprisoning large numbers of the surplus population; attributing their behaviours to individual pathology: all these cushion the rest of us from seeing how their behaviour and their drug-taking are really symptoms of the terrible way in which particular groups have been failed and abandoned as a result of major structural changes in society.

The UK government is committed to being 'tough on crime, tough on the causes of crime'. There is a growing consensus that the best way to tackle the causes of crime is to prevent criminals from offending in the first place and steer them to more profitable lifestyles. A recent Home Office study found that just 10 per cent of young offenders between the ages of 12 and 30 are responsible for nearly half the crimes committed by that age group. They are not difficult to spot in advance: truancy, exclusion from school and poor parental supervision are indicators that a child is likely to become a criminal and also a serious drug user.

In the words of one commentator:

> There is a bewildering array of initiatives aimed at tackling these problems: the Home Office £30 million 'On Track' scheme aimed at children aged between four and twelve who are at risk of getting involved in crime; a £13 million 'Youth Inclusion' programme to cut school exclusion and truancy; and a £450 million 'Children's Fund' to provide a mentoring service, education for parents and out-of-school activities … . With law enforcement officers prowling around in search of 'yobs' to curfew or fine, teenagers may well decide to seek the safety of the after-school club.[36]

Similar initiatives are taking place in most European countries.

These initiatives may well prove very effective in reducing crime in the long term, and also serious drug use. But they do not help governments to win the next election. For this purpose they must seem tough on crime itself. And this is where drug users have proved so consistently useful to politicians. Tightening drug laws wins easy applause at conferences and easy headlines in the newspapers. Unfortunately, it also exacerbates all the many worrying problems associated with drug misuse. But what's the point of a scapegoat if you can't drive it into the wilderness?

Whatever the reality behind the belief that drugs cause crime, it is difficult to see it losing its symbolic power in current circumstances. This power and endurance stems from many factors. For one thing, criminal drug users provide 'chow' for a vast host of government-employed functionaries, as a character in *The Bonfire of the Vanities* observes after watching the blue-and-orange Correction Department vans deliver felons to Bronx County Court in New York:

And to what end? ... One thing was accomplished for sure. The system was fed and these vans bought in the chow. Fifty judges, thirty-five law clerks, 245 assistant district attorneys, one DA – and Christ knows how many criminal lawyers, Legal Aid lawyers, court reporters, court clerks, court officers, correction officers, probation officers, social workers, bail bondsmen, special investigators, case clerks, court psychiatrists – what a vast swarm had to be fed! And every morning the chow came in.[37]

The idea that drugs cause crime has a reassuring simplicity and offers an endless supply of scapegoats. It provides a focus for public fears and anxieties, and an excuse for the control of the new 'dangerous classes'. It usefully masks the true economic and structural determinants of dependent drug use and acquisitive crime. It offers politicians the opportunity to court electoral popularity by appearing 'tough on crime'. Users are absolved from responsibility ('If it weren't for the gear I'd never have gone robbing'). Drug workers do not have to raise moral questions with their clients ('They have to do it'). Criminal justice agencies can wash their hands of what is seen as drug-driven crime and hand it over to treatment agencies. Treatment agencies see the carrot of more resources and feel compensated for having to dangle handcuffs in front of their patients instead of taking the old-fashioned approach of attempting to understand them. Moralists are justified in their belief that drugs are the contemporary equivalent of the plague. Liberals can argue that drug-driven crime is the consequence of prohibition and thereby push the case for legalisation.

In fact, there is some gain for all participants in the 'game' of drugs crime. As the Dodo said to Alice in Wonderland: 'Everybody has won, and all must have prizes.' Unfortunately, nobody wins in the long run because it is a Wonderland game. But a construction that has served so many separate interests for so long and that is so deeply embedded in conventional wisdom will not be easily dismantled.

Notes

1   'America bans heroin', *Bulletin on Narcotics* 5 (1953): 20–6.
2   Straw, Jack (1996) *Breaking the vicious circle: Labour's proposals to tackle drug-related crime*, London: Labour Party.
3   Marlowe, Ann (1999) *How to stop time. Heroin from A to Z*, London: Virago Press, p. 73.
4   Lindesmith, A.R. (1940) 'Dope-fiend mythology', *Journal of Criminal Issues and Criminology* 31: 179–201.

5   Courtwright, David (1982) *Dark Paradise: Opiate Addiction in America before 1940*, Cambridge, MA: Harvard University Press.

6   An exception should be made for deprived areas unfortunate enough to host 'open' drug markets, with their attendant displays of anti-social behaviour and occasional violence. Nonetheless, such effects are more properly regarded as secondary to the illegal status of drug distribution rather than directly to use of the drug.

7   Goode, E. (1993) *Drugs in American Society*, New York: McGraw-Hill.

8   For a recent example, see J. Coid and A. Carvell (2000) *The impact of methadone treatment on drug misuse and crime*, Home Office Research, Development and Statistics Directorate: Research Findings No. 12, London: Home Office.

9   For example, see M. Hough (1996) *Drug Misuse and the Criminal Justice System: a Review of the Literature*, Drug Prevention Initiative Paper 15, London: Home Office.

10 Goode (1993), p. 144.

11 Chaikin, J.M. and Chaikin, M.R. (1990) 'Drugs and predatory crime', in M. Towry and J. Wilson (eds) *Drugs and Crime*, Chicago: University of Chicago Press, pp. 203–39.

12 Gossop, M., Marsden, J. and Stewart, D. (2000) *NTORS at One Year (The National Treatment Outcome Research Study)*, London: Department of Health.

13 Personal communications from *Big Issue* vendors.

14 Ungoed-Thomas, J. and Dignan, C. (1999) 'Bootleg Britain', *Sunday Times* (7 March): 14.

15 On the political and moral uses of the heroin–crime link and for examples of statistical legerdemain from Hobson to Nixon, see the entertaining account in E.J. Epstein (1977) *Agency of Fear: Opiates and Political Power in America*, New York: G.P. Puttnam, pp. 22–45, 171–89.

16 Anthony Blair as Shadow Home Secretary. House of Commons, London: Hansard Debates (13 January 1994).

17 Blair, A. (1994) *Drugs: The Need for Action* (press release), London: Labour Party. This figure was taken from estimates produced in *Report by Greater Manchester Police Drugs & Crime Working Group* (1992).

18 See Hough (1996).

19 Dorn, N., Baker, O. and Seddon, T. (1994) *Paying for heroin: estimating the financial cost of acquisitive crime committed by dependent heroin users in England and Wales*, London: ISDD.

20 Grapendaal, M. (1992) 'Cutting their coat according to their cloth. Economic behaviour of Amsterdam opiate users', *International Journal of the Addictions* 27, 4: 487–501.

21 Mott, Joy (1981) 'Criminal involvement and penal response', in G. Edwards and C. Busch (eds) *Drug Problems in Britain*, London: Academic Press.

22 Ministry of Health (1926) *Drug Addiction: Report of the Departmental Committee on Morphine and Heroin Addiction*, London: HMSO, p. 10.

23 Bishop, Jeffrey (1957) 'Review of: Lindesmith, A. *Opiate addiction* Bloomington: Principia Press (1947)', *British Journal of Addiction* 53: 68.

24 For example, see H. Parker, R. Newcombe and K. Baxx (1988) *Living with Heroin*, Milton Keynes: Open University Press.

25 Jack Straw based his estimate on a study carried out on methadone main-
    tenance clients in Southern California between 1978–80. This study gives a
    higher figure than any other study for the proportion of addicts' income
    obtained criminally. See E. Deschenes, M. Anglin and G. Speckhart (1991)
    'Narcotics addiction: related criminal careers. Social and economic costs',
    Journal of Drug Issues 21: 383–411.
26 Grapendaal, M., Leuw, E. and Nelen, H. (1995) *A World of Opportunities*,
    New York: State University of New York Press, p. 197.
27 Bauman, Z. (1998) *Work, Consumerism and the New Poor*, Milton Keynes:
    Open University Press, p. 74.
28 See Advisory Council for the Misuse of Drugs (1998) *Drug Misuse and the
    Environment*, London: HMSO.
29 Bruce Johnson and colleagues provided a different view, based on one of
    the most detailed and methodologically sophisticated studies of the
    heroin–crime link in New York in the 1980s. They pointed out some of the
    economic advantages deprived neighbourhoods gained from the presence
    of a large number of addict criminals and the accompanying informal
    economy that develops around this. Non-drug users in such communities
    are able to access stolen goods they could not have afforded. He described
    housewives waiting on the doorsteps for the cheap joints of meat to be
    delivered from the hustling expeditions.
        He also argued that the thefts of heroin users might bring some
    economic benefit for wider society because they increase the monetary
    wealth in the formal economy. Victims buy replacements for the goods
    they have had stolen, shops transfer shoplifting losses to customers and
    the government gains added sales-tax revenue. We are not economists, but
    we find this part of the argument dubious. See B. Johnson *et al.* (1985)
    Taking Care of Business: the Economics of Crime by Heroin Abusers,
    Lexington: D.C. Heath.
30 Stimson, Gerry (2000) *The Unhealthy State of British Drugs Policy*, speech
    delivered at Methadone Alliance Conference, London, 22 March.
31 Drug law is generally bizarre. According to present interpretations,
    handing round a joint is not supplying, nor is leaving a joint with a friend
    while you go to get a drink. But if the friend gives it back to you later, then
    he is deemed guilty of supplying. For these and other niceties, see Rudi
    Fortson (1992) *The Law on the Misuse of Drugs and Drug Trafficking
    Offences*, London : Sweet & Maxwell.
32 *Time* (30 June 1980), quoted in Arnold Trebach, 'The Lessons of
    Ayatollah Khalkhali', *Journal of Drug Issues* (1981): 391–2.
33 Belenko, Steven (1998) *Behind Bars: Substance Abuse and America's Prison
    Population*, New York: National Center on Addiction and Substance
    Abuse, Columbia University.
34 Christie, N. (2000) *Crime Control as Industry: Towards a Western System of
    Gulags*, London: Routledge, p. 68.
35 Gordon, Diana (1994) *The Return of the Dangerous Classes: Drug
    Prohibition and Policy Politics*, New York: Norton.
36 Miles, Alice (2000) 'Curfews and fines won't stop youth crimes', *The Times*
    (7 December): 22.
37 Wolfe, Tom (1988) *The Bonfire of the Vanities*, London: Jonathan Cape,
    p. 40.

7   *The hardest drug or the gentle drug*

Heroin and health

The Hardest Drug: Heroin and public policy
                                    Title of book by John Kaplan[1]

'Heroin: the gentle drug'
                                    Title of article by Dale Beckett[2]

Heroin can be used as a medicine or as a drug of addiction or, indeed, as a means of obtaining occasional pleasure in the way that many people have a drink at weekends. But because people think of it as a 'drug', they often think it can only be harmful and unhealthy. Medical substances have numerous and variable effects, which can be put to good or harmful use. For this reason, doctors and pharmacists use the word 'drug' in a different sense from the public. A drug is any chemical or herbal substance that can be used to produce an effect on body function. Aspirin, ginseng and heroin are therefore all drugs. It does not matter whether or not they cause dependency or are abused by addicts, or whether the effects are predominantly harmful or beneficial.

This used to be the normal meaning of the word. A drugstore was where one bought medicines and a druggist was a pharmacist. During this century the word 'drug' has taken on sinister connotations. It now tends to mean for most people the kind of nasty stuff that is taken by drug addicts, in other words something harmful and dangerous. This can cause confusion when discussing a particular substance such as heroin. In truth it is a 'drug' in the medical sense, but there is much more to it than its notorious role as a potential drug of addiction.

The distinction becomes clear when we compare it to its close relative, morphine. The effects of the two medications are extremely similar, as indeed are all the drugs of the opiate family. But whereas heroin has developed a reputation for evil, morphine is generally perceived as a beneficial medicine.

In fact, both substances are extremely good medicines. As relatives of opium, they belong to that family which has been rightly valued from time immemorial as the supreme painkillers.

> Among the remedies which it has pleased Almighty God to give man to relieve his sufferings, none is so universal and so efficacious as opium.[3]

This view, expressed by the seventeenth-century physician Thomas Sydenham, is still true today. Opiates remain the most effective analgesics and if they were all abolished from medical use there would be a huge increase in human suffering. They are also useful in a number of other conditions, including diarrhoea, heart failure and intractable cough.

They are both 'gentle' drugs because they can be taken for long periods without causing physical harm. But they are also both 'hard' drugs because they can lead to addiction, to self-destructive behaviour and to death by overdose.

Addiction will be considered in detail in Chapter 8, but there is ample evidence that the risks of dependence are small when opiates are used for pain relief rather than self-gratification. In one study, the files were examined of 11,882 consecutive hospital patients who had received opiate medication for pain. Only four of these developed any kind of addictive problem and in only one was it considered serious.[4] Nonetheless, exaggerated fears of addiction have made doctors nervous about prescribing opiates in adequate doses. Even dying patients are often denied proper relief of suffering, apparently for fear of inducing addiction. It is hard to understand why morphine or heroin dependence during terminal illness should be considered a serious problem even if it did develop. Nonetheless, it has become such a strong anxiety among prescribing doctors that the term 'opiophobia' has been coined, meaning an irrational fear of using effective amounts of opiate analgesic. It is clearly not just the public which has been misled by the connotations of 'drug use'.

In fact, heroin causes little physical harm and may be taken over long periods with safety. This may surprise those who have read alarmist anti-drugs propaganda. It is true that many heroin users become ill, but this is usually the result of using contaminated injecting equipment or impure supplies of the drug.[5] In this way they develop abscesses and thromboses, hepatitis and HIV infection.[6] All this would be avoided if they had ready access to clean equipment and pharmaceutical heroin.

Heroin use in pregnancy may lead to low-weight babies, but this effect is hard to disentangle from all the other causes of low birth-weight which are common in heroin users, such as poor diet, alcohol and nicotine misuse.

In general, heroin has little adverse effect on health. A hundred years ago the Royal Commission on Opium concluded that opium was a safe drug when used in moderation: 'we have no hesitation in saying that no extended physical or moral degradation is caused by the habit'.[7] A large study at Philadelphia General Hospital during the 1920s showed that this was also true of heroin. In all, 861 male addicts (80 per cent of them addicted to heroin and the rest to morphine or other opiates) participated in various phases of this study. The medical research team organised exhaustive tests and observations. Their conclusions were clear:

> the study shows that morphine addiction is not characterized by physical deterioration or impairment of physical fitness aside from the addiction per se. There is no evidence of change in the circulatory, hepatic, renal or endocrine functions. When it is considered that these subjects had been addicted for at least five years, some of them for as long as twenty years, these negative observations are highly significant.[8]

This opinion is echoed in a recent expert review: 'Apart from these effects [tolerance and withdrawal] there is little evidence that long-term use of heroin is damaging to health.'[9]

For these reasons, many physicians have argued that heroin should be readily available for medical use, and have resisted its gradual disappearance and the increasing restrictions on its use. A basic knowledge of the pharmacology of heroin is necessary to understand the arguments for and against its use as a medicine. In particular, it is important to appreciate in what respects it differs from morphine, which is still considered a useful medicine throughout the world.

The pharmacology of opioids[10]

Heroin is an opioid, which means that it is closely related to medications derived from the opium poppy, such as morphine and codeine. Opioids influence the body by reacting with specific opioid receptors found on the surface of cells, particularly in those areas of the brain and spinal cord associated with mood control and the perception of pain. These are designed principally to react to internal, or 'endogenous', opioids, which are produced by the body itself as a form of chemical messenger. There are three main types of endogenous opioid: endorphins, enkephalins and dynorphins. There are also three main types of opioid receptor, named mu-, kappa- and delta-receptors.

Unfortunately for the student, it is not the case that each type of internal opioid reacts with one type of receptor. The reactions are far more complicated and still not well understood. Each opioid reacts to a different extent at each type of receptor and each type of receptor may produce different physiological results according to its situation in the body. Moreover, new receptor subtypes are still being discovered. Opioid receptor chemistry is an exciting area of contemporary brain research, which fortunately does not require detailed elucidation in the present discussion.

Like most medicines, opioids therefore work by imitating an internal process of the body. The families of chemicals produced by plants, animals and other organisms are limited. We all stem from the same ancestors and share many genes in common. These genes manufacture similar chemicals, but they are used for different purposes in different organisms.

It is perhaps a coincidence that chemical messengers controlling pain in the human brain are so like those produced by opium poppies.[11] On the other hand, poppies and humans have lived so closely together for so long that some form of symbiotic evolution may have occurred. Humans were more likely to cultivate poppies containing high amounts of opium. This is a normal process in plant breeding. More interestingly, those of our ancestors who responded most strongly to the pain-relieving qualities of opium may thereby have acquired some competitive advantage in the battle for survival. In this way, humans and poppies may gradually have each acquired characteristics advantageous to the other.

Activation of opiate receptors does not just affect mood and perception of pain. Morphine and heroin are opiates that work primarily at mu-receptors. Mu-receptor activation also has important effects on the eyes, the vomiting centre and the balancing mechanism, the blood vessels, the lungs and the respiratory system, the digestive system, the bladder, the womb, the skin and the immune system. There are many varieties of opiate, but morphine is the one most similar to heroin. As morphine is also in general medical use, it is the opiate most useful to compare with heroin.

The eye provides the most visible indication of opiate use. Constriction of the pupil gives the typical 'pinned eyes' of the opiate addict. This is one of the few opiate effects which does not diminish with prolonged use as a result of tolerance. It is almost unknown to see large pupils after heroin use or small ones during withdrawal. Opiates also lower the fluid pressure in the eyeball, which may be of benefit in glaucoma.

Opiates often produce nausea and vomiting. For the most part this only occurs when the subject is standing. It results from direct stimulation of the vomiting centre in the brain, combined with an effect on the balancing mechanism in the ear. This effect is probably more marked with morphine than with heroin. Doctors have therefore found heroin a useful alternative in pain control if patients become nauseous after taking morphine.

Mu-stimulation also produces relaxation of blood vessels and a reduction in the normal reflexes which maintain blood pressure. This effect is slight in normal subjects, but can be very useful in acute heart failure, for example after a heart attack. The injection of morphine or heroin reduces the workload of the heart by reducing the resistance of the circulation. It also brings mental relief at a time of great anxiety. Where available, heroin is used in preference to morphine because of its quicker onset of action. It is still used regularly in the UK for the immediate treatment of heart attack.

There are a number of effects on the digestive system. The main effect is to slow down the activity of the stomach and bowel. As a result, more fluid is absorbed from the faeces and they become hard and difficult to pass. Constipation is a regular complaint of opiate users, both addicts and those being treated for pain. However, it is more of a problem with morphine than with heroin. The reason for this lies in the easier absorption of heroin across the blood/brain barrier. Less heroin is needed to produce appropriate pain control or mood modulation, and there is proportionately less effect on the bowel. Conversely, morphine is widely used to treat diarrhoea. In this case, mental effects are not required and so poor absorption into the brain is an advantage.

After injection of morphine, the pressure in the bile tract increases for about two hours and the valve, or sphincter, that controls bile release may go into spasm. This may be bad enough to cause biliary colic and can certainly exacerbate biliary colic if it is given mistakenly to help the pain. Heroin is less active in this regard. For this reason, surgeons used to prefer heroin for pain relief after bile-duct surgery. More recently developed opioids such as fentanyl and nalbuphine have much less bile-duct activity than heroin or morphine, and this is therefore no longer a particular reason to use heroin.

Both heroin and morphine reduce activity to some extent in the uterus and bladder, but this improves with the development of tolerance. Both may be associated with some slight reduction in immune system activity, but it is debatable whether this has any real effect in making users more liable to develop infections. Both also can cause flushing and itching in the skin due to the release of histamine. This is much more marked with morphine than with heroin and may cause some patients to give up morphine treatment.

They are also very effective in reducing uncomfortable coughing. This was a major advantage in the treatment of tuberculosis. Nowadays, they have been replaced by related drugs which are non-addictive but equally effective in suppressing the cough reflex. These include dextromorphan and pholcodeine, often found in proprietary cough medicines.

It can be seen therefore that heroin has possible application to a number of medical conditions and that, in some circumstances, it has advantages over morphine. On the whole it is a gentle drug, causing pleasant sensations and little physical harm. No one can deny its hard side, most strikingly revealed by the ever-increasing toll of overdose death. But it can be argued that this is not a problem inherent in the drug, but a consequence of the type of people who tend to use it under present social conditions. Morphine is equally dangerous in overdose and indeed was a common cause of overdose death in the last century.

Overdose

Overdose is the commonest cause of death for heroin addicts. The frequency of overdose in this group has increased in Britain by a factor of eight over the last ten years and is rapidly approaching road-deaths as the most frequent cause of death among young people. Overdose has also increased at an alarming rate in the US, where heroin users attending casualty doubled from 34,000 to 70,000 between 1990 and 1996.

Heroin deaths disproportionately affect deprived areas, with those from the lowest social class being six times as likely to die as those from the highest class. It occurs almost exclusively among injectors, who thereby have a mortality rate about fifteen times higher than the average for their age. There are areas of our inner cities where everybody knows families who have lost members to drug overdose. The numbers of deaths are small when compared to those due to alcohol and smoking,[12] but they are particularly tragic because they occur among the young and with disproportionate frequency in certain areas. You would be ill advised to argue that heroin was a gentle drug in the poorer areas of Dublin and Glasgow.

In North Dublin, for example, so many young people have died in this way that local families have commissioned a sculpture in their memory. It will stand on a traffic island that was once a notorious centre for drug dealing. Sculptor Leo Higgins is reproducing in Irish limestone the hallway of a typical Dublin terrace house. The door will be half open, revealing a flame of gilded bronze to 'keep alive memories of home, where those who are gone are never forgotten'.[13] In this way families hope to reclaim this territory for their community. With its echoes of a war memorial the design of the sculpture underlines the pathos of this contemporary scourge. They may not be 'glorious dead', but their lost lives are equally tragic.

However, most of these deaths are readily preventable. The real tragedy is that the deaths are needless. Drug users have only recently started receiving courses on first aid and proper advice about how to avoid overdose. Effective prevention must also depend on a good understanding of the common circumstances of death. This must be communicated to people who use drugs. They must also be reassured that seeking medical aid will not lead to prosecution. Too many people die without any proper attempt to save them.

Heroin overdose interferes with the control of respiration. The breathing reflex is complicated, but is principally driven by a brain centre that reacts to rising amounts of carbon dioxide in the blood. The process of breathing brings oxygen into the system and expels carbon dioxide, the unwanted result of cell metabolism. As carbon dioxide levels rise, the breathing centre kicks in and triggers another breath. This automatic process is interrupted by large doses of morphine or heroin. At a certain level of overdose, patients may breathe only when instructed to do so. Beyond this, coma ensues and then death from respiratory failure.

Regular users acquire considerable tolerance to this process. It has been shown that they can safely tolerate up to nine times their standard dose. In an early study, three addicts were given six, seven and nine times their customary doses intravenously. Far from causing death, the drug 'resulted in insignificant changes in the pulse and respiration rates, electrocardiogram, chemical studies of the blood, and the behaviour of the addict'. They did not even become drowsy.[14]

You might think therefore that overdoses occurred for the most part in naïve users with little experience or tolerance, who had perhaps got hold of the drug for the first time at a party. In fact, this is not the case. The majority of victims are in their late twenties or early thirties and have used heroin for at least twelve years. They are almost exclusively injectors. Most will have been present at the death of other users and will themselves have experienced many previous non-fatal over-doses. For the most part they have never been in treatment and only rarely are they in treatment at the time of death. A small but significant group have recently been released from prison.

Usually heroin is taken alongside other drugs, particularly alcohol and tranquillisers. For the most part, morphine levels in the blood at post-mortem[15] are no higher than in heroin addicts who have died of other causes, for example violence or accident. Drug impurities are often blamed, but rarely make any contribution. Some authorities have questioned the role of quinine, which is sometimes an ingredient of street heroin. In fact, quinine is rarely found outside the US and even there is not found in toxic concentrations.[16]

Most fatal overdoses occur in company, but in most cases companions do not seek medical help. Instead they are liable to try a number of home-made resuscitation techniques of dubious worth. In one study, the most used methods were sticking a twig down the throat, jumping up and down with the victim on one's back or bumping them rapidly down the stairs. If all else failed, they would take the victim out into the street and leave them there in the hope that somebody might find them and ring a taxi. Almost never did their companions follow the recommended approach, namely to place the victim in recovery position and ring an ambulance.[17]

What does all this mean? In a few cases, heroin overdose is a result of poor tolerance. For the most part, this occurs when users come out of prison and decide to celebrate, but forget that they have lost their tolerance. Although drugs are commonplace in prisons nowadays, very few inmates use as much as they did outside prison. If they revert straightaway to their former pattern of use, overdose is a real risk. This could be prevented by proper education of prisoners and their relatives before release.

Occasionally, death occurs in naïve users. A vigorous public education campaign is required to ensure that everybody knows that small amounts of heroin and methadone can be fatal if the body is not used to them. This is particularly so if the drugs are given to children. Every year one or two deaths of children occur when parents out of ignorance have given them a little methadone to help them settle. Successful education campaigns have been carried out in the past about the dangers of drugs like paracetamol and now everybody knows that too much paracetamol can kill you.

In the majority of cases, heroin is not in itself the cause of death, but only in combination with alcohol and tranquillisers. The combination causes death because people take it in a reckless manner. In spite of numerous warnings from their own experience, they continue to dice with death by using excessive amounts of all three types of drug.[18] The risk of death may even confer a perverse glamour. US dealers often enhance the appeal of their product by using trade names such as 'body bag', 'no mercy', 'homicide' and 'silver bullet'.[19] Comedian Lenny Bruce was asked whether he would die young as a result of his heroin habit. He replied 'Yeah – but I can't explain – it's like kissing God.'[20] Too many users share his view.

This is perhaps not surprising, because heroin is a marginalised drug. It is taken mostly by people on the fringes of society and by people who are by nature risk-takers. Users also include a high percentage of people who suffer from mental illness, particularly depression and personality disorder. They are often poor at estimating danger and taking 'avoiding action'. In one study, most people who had been treated for overdose-induced coma did not judge that they were at risk in future, even though most of them had had several similar previous experiences. Moreover, the majority of them were not interested in enlisting for treatment.

Fortunately, heroin overdose is very treatable. A drug called naloxone blocks the action of heroin and produces rapid recovery. It is very important to persuade users to call an ambulance as soon as a companion becomes unconscious. This will only happen if there is a concerted effort by police, doctors and ambulance staff to reassure users that they will not be liable for prosecution or even have their names taken if they contact emergency services in these circumstances. It will also be helpful if drug users have better knowledge about the dangers of mixing drugs and the principles of first aid. Drug workers are only just beginning to realise how useful training courses in prison can be in spreading this knowledge among the drug-using community.

At present, trials of take-home naloxone are being carried out. It is hoped that with proper training users will be able to administer this opiate antagonist to companions in an emergency and thus reverse the physical effects of overdose. This will be easier when it becomes available as a nasal spray. It remains to be seen whether this will lead to lives being saved or have a paradoxical effect of encouraging more dangerous drug use because users believe that they will now have a chemical 'airbag' if things go wrong.[21] It has even been suggested that some may use naloxone spray as a weapon, by threatening other addicts with instant withdrawal at the press of a button. However, this is a trial well worth the effort. A reversal of the ever-upward trend of heroin deaths would be a considerable achievement.

Or perhaps whisky and biscuits would work just as well. The first recorded overdose comes from a personal account by a doctor in 1901:

> I took an overdose of heroin, estimated at about 1.5 grain [100 mg], not knowing the amount. Shortly afterwards I began to feel a tingling all over and things appeared a little different to what they should be. I felt intense sleepiness coming on, and at once went out and harnessed my horse and commenced to drive country-wards to keep in the open. I reached a farmhouse a mile or two distant and took a cup of tea and a biscuit, feeling unwell. They also gave me a quarter of a glass of whisky to which I added some warm water. I returned home at the end of two hours, and attended to two patients. I lay down afterwards, and at the end of six hours was able to feel free of all danger of falling asleep.[22]

The medical retreat from heroin

Although nobody now shares the same enthusiasm for heroin as its initial advocates, the medical retreat from heroin is not a result of the development of better medicines, but an unfortunate side effect of the world wide campaign against drug addiction.

When heroin was first released, doctors welcomed it as another weapon in the fight against tuberculosis. TB has recently made some-thing of a comeback, but for many years it almost vanished. Few now appreciate the fear that the disease aroused or the misery it caused to sufferers. Until the arrival of effective antibiotics in the early 1950s, the 'white plague' worked on the public imagination like cancer and AIDS combined. Doctors were understandably enthusiastic about any new medication that could relieve the distress of sufferers. The case of Miss M was typical:

> Miss M, 22 years old, was admitted for pleurisy with effusion, with incipient pulmonary TB, July 26th 1898. Her chief complaint was a hard dry cough, which caused her great distress, especially at night. Codeine afforded no relief. Heroin, a sixth of a grain, relieved it within half an hour; when given at night, she slept about six hours without coughing.[23]

At first it was thought that heroin had a specific stimulant effect on respiration. It was claimed that 'it allows lengthening and deepening of breathing, so the blood oxygen is better'.[24] Later it was firmly established that this was not the case; in fact just the opposite.[25]

Heroin reduces respiratory rate and volume, and thus also the blood oxygen concentration. Why did good doctors get this wrong? There were perhaps two reasons.

The recent discovery of the specific stimulatory effect of digitalis on the heart had prepared medical minds to look for a medicine with a similar effect on respiration. The effect on patients was more persuasive still. Patients with severe cough and shortness of breath, like Miss M, were undoubtedly very frightened and uncomfortable. Perhaps a portion of their rapid breathing was due to anxiety rather than just to the poor condition of their lungs. Heroin slowed down the breathing rate and this in itself made patients calmer, even if it did not help their oxygen levels. It is also very effective in suppressing troublesome coughing. On top of this, it is matchless in producing a mental state of calm detachment. Patients remain aware of their pain and illness, but no longer feel it really matters. Much of the horror of illness lies in the fear it induces. Miss M slept well because she coughed less, her breathing pattern was less disruptive and she felt less frightened.

Even many decades later, when doctors had accepted that it did not cause respiratory stimulation, they still found it useful in terminal tuberculosis:

> During this final stage [of consumption] heroin, by calming the distressing sensation of asphyxia, soothing the cough and leaving room for hope, can still be used as a valuable medicament which can soothe when all others have ceased to be effective.

The same writer also found it invaluable for patients dying of heart failure, when 'it relieves anginal pain, insomnia, extreme distress and difficulty in breathing'.[26]

Ironically, this was written shortly before the United States banned the use of heroin as a medicine altogether through the Narcotic Control Act of 1956[27] and indeed before its medicinal use disappeared in all but a handful of countries. Between 1928 and 1930 two tons of licit heroin had been consumed annually across the world, ostensibly for medicinal purposes. By 1959 the situation had changed radically. Forty kilograms were consumed in the United Kingdom, seven kilograms in Belgium, three in France, one each in Paraguay and Portugal, and almost none anywhere else.[28] By the early 1980s British doctors were writing just under 99 per cent of the world's prescriptions for medicinal heroin.[29] Of other countries Belgium alone continued to allow its use.[30]

This eclipse of medicinal heroin did not occur because more effective drugs had superseded it or because it had been shown to be ineffective in medical trials. It disappeared principally because of America's experience of heroin addiction and consequent pressure from its diplomats transmitted through the International Narcotics Control Board (INCB). In 1956 even the United Kingdom bowed to pressure and announced its intention to ban heroin. This followed a call from the INCB to 'fulfil a humanitarian task, which is in keeping with its traditions'.[31]

In the event, this decision was resisted and overturned by British doctors, who did not see why they should abandon a useful medicine. In one contemporary survey, the surgeons consulted 'were all supporters of diamorphine'. It was particularly useful for 'pain relief after biliary operations'. It was excellent for cough, 'especially cancer and influenza'.[32] It was essential for pain relief 'in the fifteen percent of patients who are always very sick after morphine'.[33] Many were sceptical anyway that a medicinal ban would be effective in preventing the spread of addiction. One eminent physician spoke for many when he argued that heroin use would probably increase after a ban, 'because it would be made worthwhile for professional peddlers'.[32]

In America there were many physicians and members of the public who wished to see heroin restored to the Pharmacopoeia. In the words of one cancer specialist,

> Right now, in America, we know of a drug which is the most potent, effective, soluble and rapidly active narcotic ever created. It is not available. I do not understand this.[34]

The National Committee on Treatment of Intractable Pain was formed in 1977 to lobby for the use of heroin, particularly in terminal illness. It was headed by the redoubtable Judith Quattelbaum, who claimed that about 40,000 Americans were dying every year with pain that did not respond to available analgesics. The case was also put with force by a professor of law, Dr Arnold Trebach, who carried out a number of fact-finding missions to Britain and wrote an influential book based on his findings.[35]

Although the Department of Health and Human Services and the Drug Enforcement Agency resisted the reinstatement of heroin, it received sympathetic consideration from many politicians. The issue roused considerable passion, perhaps predictably because it linked cancer, the most feared disease, with heroin, the most feared drug. Officials claimed that there was little research evidence to support a case for change. But, as Congressman Neal argued,

We need more study, but to get the study, we need a substance available for you to study. But as long as it's under Schedule 1, it will not be available, because the assumption will be that there is no medical use. It's a Catch-22 situation, it seems to me.[36]

In effect, this version of Catch-22 has inhibited the rational consideration of heroin's use as medicine ever since. Doctors have avoided research in this contentious area or have been prevented by local legislation. Fortunately, this has started to change very recently with regard to the use of heroin for the treatment of drug dependence. We will return to this in Chapter 8.

In the event, the United States government permitted two research studies into the use of heroin in terminal care. One study at Georgetown Medical Center indicated that heroin had some advantages over morphine. It was more potent and therefore smaller quantities could be administered. This was helpful in patients with wasted muscles who could not tolerate frequent large injections. Onset of relief was more rapid and it appeared to provide a more euphoric feeling. The other study at Memorial Sloane Kettering was less favourable. It did not establish any specific advantages over morphine, but reported that pain relief and euphoria were less well maintained than with morphine.

These equivocal results did little to settle the debate. Many continued to believe that an increase in medicinal use would lead to increased illegal consumption. But, as one congressman remarked,

Four point three illegal tons of heroin are brought into this country each year, in other words the weight of two elephants. Medical use for dying patients would be a pimple on the posterior of one of those elephants.[34]

Eventually, the House subcommittee charged with considering the issue proposed to Congress the Compassionate Pain Relief Act, which would allow the use of heroin in terminal illness. In the words of its chairman, 'It is time for Congress ... to offer a new perception of a compassionate, balanced and hopeful drug policy for this nation.'[37]

The Compassionate Pain Relief Act was defeated in 1985 and has not been reconsidered since. The combined influence of the Department of Health and the Drug Enforcement Agency proved too powerful, along with the spectre they raised of uncontrolled heroin addiction. The influence of the US has been such that no other country has seriously considered reintroducing medicinal heroin until the recent Swiss experiments. Only British doctors have continued to prescribe heroin, but even in Britain its use has become slightly apologetic and surreptitious. Other drugs are preferred where possible, not for medical reasons but perhaps because of qualms concerning its evil reputation.

Pain control

The most important medicinal use for heroin and other opioids is in the treatment of severe pain. For a long time heroin was a standard component of the famous 'Brompton Cocktail', first devised by Herbert Snow at the Brompton Hospital at the turn of the last century for the treatment of terminal pain. Initially this cocktail contained heroin or morphine, cocaine and sometimes also small amounts of alcohol. The heroin and alcohol provided calmness and analgesia, while the cocaine preserved alertness. It remained a standard treatment in many hospitals for over eighty years.

A review was published in 1974 of 500 patients with advanced malignancy treated with oral heroin/cocaine mixture or with heroin injection if they were unable to take medicine by mouth. Most patients were able to continue on the oral medication at least until the last two days before death. The cocaine dose was kept constant at 10 mg/day, while the heroin was adjusted either upwards or downwards each day according to how much was needed to control pain. It was found that for most patients the required dose reached a plateau which could be maintained, in other words that it did not keep increasing. No withdrawal symptoms were noted on dose reduction. The authors concluded that tolerance was not a practical problem, even over a period of six months. They also did not observe any development of dependence or addiction. In particular they were impressed by the cocktail because there was 'no impairment of mental faculties'.[38]

This was also prized by Dr Elizabeth Kubler-Ross, who used the cocktail extensively alongside her psychotherapeutic work with dying patients at the Methodist Hospital of Indiana. Her prescription contained morphine and cocaine, because heroin was outlawed by the American regulations.[39] She described with great clarity the process of mental adjustment that needs to take place in people approaching death. Typical stages *en route* include periods of denial, of angry rejection and of depressed submission. She believed that patients and their relatives often needed help in understanding these normal reactions and in moving through them so that death could ultimately be faced with some measure of acceptance. Her work has been very influential in the hospice movement and also among psychotherapists dealing with other forms of loss, such as bereavement, where similar mental reactions often occur.

Kubler-Ross believed that proper pain control was essential in this process, provided mental alertness could also be maintained. Opiates such as morphine and heroin have a unique role in severe pain. Not only do they remove pain, but they also allow a sense of personal detachment from the pain while maintaining the ability to communicate and think clearly. They are not used in order to get high or escape from reality, but as a way of confronting with dignity the challenge of illness and death.

In fact, it became clear with further trials that diamorphine was the critical component in the cocktail and that cocaine did little to increase alertness, but was responsible sometimes for restlessness, depression and even hallucinations.[40] The mixture was often made up with gin, whisky or brandy. Apart from providing a certain bohemian cheer during a difficult time, it also preserved the mixture for longer. Diamorphine powder dissolves well in alcohol and will then keep its efficacy for up to six months.[41]

Heroin has some advantage over morphine in terminal pain relief. It is more concentrated, so less is needed; this is particularly helpful when injections have to be given. It is less likely to produce nausea and itching. It also gets into the brain more quickly, although with regular use this advantage ceases to be relevant. It remains the drug of choice in the UK when subcutaneous treatment is required.[42] It is for this reason that there has been pressure from physicians in many countries to bring heroin back onto their formularies. In fact, with the development of newer opioids such as fentanyl and new techniques such as continuous subcutaneous morphine infusion, there is no longer any definite need for diamorphine: other drugs can do the job almost as well. On the other hand, the other opioids are equally addictive and no more efficacious. On any fair assessment, one would have to say that, even after a hundred years, heroin remains a medicine without superior.

In the 1970s one of the main protagonists of heroin use in terminal care was a British physician named Dr Robert Twycross. Although he described heroin as 'an indispensable, potent, narcotic analgesic',[38] he later disappointed Arnold Trebach by not supporting his campaign to reintroduce heroin into American cancer wards. Dr Trebach accepted this philosophically 'as part of the often conflicted nature of the field'.[35] The reason Dr Twycross did not support the campaign is interesting and important. He argued that 'the doctors who use their present narcotics badly will use heroin just as badly, and, in practice, patients will be no better off'.[30] Later he wrote that

> the availability of heroin would not correct the tragic inadequacy of pain control endemic in North American hospitals. The important factor is not choice of narcotic but adequate scheduling.[43]

The truth was that patients were not receiving sufficient doses of opiates as often as they needed them. The more tragic truth is that for most of the world this is still the case. The techniques of pain control have developed hugely, particularly in specialised enclaves such as hospices for palliative care. Nonetheless, two-thirds of patients dying of cancer are likely to suffer chronic severe pain before they die. The fear of heroin has contaminated doctors' perception of the other opiates, such as morphine, and their reluctance to use them is just as strong.

The situation is so serious that the International Narcotics Control Board has recently taken upon itself the task of providing guidance on the proper use of opiates. We make no apology for quoting at length from its recent publication:

> In spite of recent progress, the medical use and availability of opioid analgesics continue to be relatively moderate. In a large proportion of the countries and territories in the world, insignificant amounts of these medicines are available for medical purposes and it is generally agreed that the treatment of chronic or acute pain caused by cancer is still inadequate: only about 10–30 per cent of patients may be receiving adequate treatment, even in many technologically advanced countries. The rate is much lower in developing countries ... . The 10 largest consumer countries accounted for as much as 80 per cent of analgesic morphine consumption. The average per capita consumption of morphine in 1998 in the 10 countries with the highest morphine consumption levels was 31 grams per 1,000 inhabitants. In the 10 countries with the next highest consumption levels, the corresponding figure was 16 grams per 1,000 inhabitants. In the next 60 countries, with a total morphine consumption of more than 1 kg, it was only 2 grams per 1,000 inhabitants. In the remaining 120 countries, there was little or no opioid consumption. Several African countries reported no morphine consumption. The most frequently mentioned causes of inadequate opioid availability are restrictive regulations, cumbersome administrative procedures, concerns

about diversion and the consequences of inadvertent errors, concerns about iatrogenic addiction, and inadequate or insufficient training of health personnel.[44]

The INCB must be commended for its campaign. But unfortunately the restrictive regulations and cumbersome procedures are almost entirely a result of its earlier work and that of its predecessors. Throughout history even the poorest have had access to the God-given benefits of the poppy. As a result of the eighty years' war against heroin, there are now 120 countries where nobody receives this relief at all, even when undergoing the severest pain. The extent of human suffering is incalculable. Heroin is now readily available in the back-streets of Glasgow or Manchester for £10 a wrap, but denied to people throughout the world who are suffering the agonies of terminal cancer.

What is uncertain is whether a change can be brought about in the practice of health authorities and prescribing physicians without a sea change in our attitudes to heroin and a realisation that, as well as being a drug of addiction, it is also an excellent medicine. Until this happens, its evil reputation will inevitably contaminate our attitudes to other opiates. Like heroin, they can all lead to addiction when used for pleasure. But many physicians continue to ignore the compelling evidence that they are extremely unlikely to lead to addiction when used in the treatment of severe pain.

Notes

1   Kaplan, John (1983) *The Hardest Drug: Heroin and public policy*, Chicago: University of Chicago Press.
2   Beckett, H. Dale (1979) 'Heroin: the gentle drug', *New Society* (26 July), pp, 181–2.
3   Sydenham, Thomas (1742) quoted in Berridge, V and Edwards, G (1987) *Opium and the People,* New Haven: Yale University, p. xxiv.
4   Porter, J. and Jick, H. (1980) 'Addiction rare in patients treated with narcotics', *New England Journal of Medicine* 302: 123. For a review of this issue, see World Health Organisation (1990) *Cancer pain relief and palliative care: Report of a WHO Expert Committee*, Geneva: WHO. They conclude that 'the medical use of opiates is rarely associated with the development of psychological dependence'.
5   There is a rare condition called leucoencephalopathy. This is a progressive brain disease which leads rapidly to coma and death. It has been observed occasionally in heroin users who chase the dragon (see E.C. Wolters, F.C. Stam and R.J. Lousberg (1982) 'Leucoencephalopathy after inhaling "heroin" pyrolysate', *Lancet* 2: 1,233–7). The cause is uncertain, but is most likely due to an abnormal contaminant, perhaps noscapine which can produce toxic fumes when burnt with ascorbic acid (see H. Huizer (1987)

'Analytical studies on illicit heroin. V. Efficacy of volatilisation during heroin smoking', *Pharmaceutish Weekblad (Scientific Edition)* 9: 203–11).

6   A recent batch of infected heroin led to a number of deaths among injectors in the UK and Ireland. The causative organism was probably *Clostridium novyi*, which is rare in humans but a common cause of animal disease. One disease it causes is the dreaded Black Disease in goats, described succinctly in a standard veterinary manual: '*Symptoms*: a dead goat. *Treatment*: bury very deep or burn the carcase.' See Max Merrall (2000) *The A–Z of goat diseases*, http://www.caprine.co.nz/reference/ 01goat_diseases.htm. Tragically, the infection was equally devastating in heroin users. At least thirty young people died within days of injecting contaminated supplies. Had thirty people died of contaminated beer, there would have been calls for a public enquiry and it would have been dubbed a national disaster. The deaths of the heroin users passed without comment.

7   *Royal Commission on Opium*, London: British Parliamentary Papers (1894–95).

8   Light, A.B. and Torrance, E.G. (1929) 'The effect of abrupt withdrawal followed by administration of morphine in heroin addicts', *Archives of Internal Medicine* 44: 870–6.

9   Working Party for Royal Colleges of Psychiatrists and Physicians (2000) *Drugs – Choices and Dilemmas*, London: Gaskell Press, p. 15.

10 This account is principally indebted to the various editions of Goodman and Gilman's *Pharmacological Basis of Therapeutics*, New York: McGraw-Hill. In particular, Jerome Jaffe and William Martin's excellent account of 'Opioid analgesics and antagonists' in the 8th edition has not been fully superseded by later editions.

11 The resemblance is closer in some mammals. For example, the liver of the rat synthesises morphine naturally. See C.J. Weitz, K.F. Faull and A. Goldstein (1987) 'Synthesis of the skeleton of the morphine molecule by mammalian liver', *Nature* 330: 674–7.

12 In the UK it is reckoned that there about 2,000 deaths due to drug overdose per year, 40,000 as a result of alcohol abuse and 120,000 as a result of smoking. The number of drug-related deaths is bound to rise as a result of chronic infection. Of injecting drug users, 70 per cent are infected with Hepatitis C. Of these, 80 per cent will develop chronic infection, of which 20 per cent are likely to die of cirrhosis or liver cancer. This probably amounts to about 7,000 to 8,000 of current users, but this number could be reduced dramatically if sufferers receive appropriate treatment.

13 Birchard, K. (1999) 'Remembering those who died from heroin addiction', *Lancet* 354: 9,176.

14 Light, A.B. and Torrance, E.G. (1929) 'The effect of intramuscular and intravenous injection of large doses of morphine to heroin addicts', *Archives of Internal Medicine* 44: 376–94.

15 You will remember that heroin breaks down rapidly in the body to morphine.

16 Darke, S. and Zador, D. (1996) 'Fatal heroin "overdose": a review', *Addiction* 91: 1,765–72.

17 Hardman, J. (1996) 'An Exploration of Drug Users' Attendance and Non-attendance at Accident and Emergency Departments', M.Sc. thesis, Manchester.

18 Sporer, K.A. (1999) 'Acute heroin overdose', *Annals of Internal Medicine* 130, 7: 584–90.

19 M (1994) 'Listening to heroin', *Village Voice*: 25–30.

20 Krassner, Paul (2000) 'The last laugh. The busting of Lenny Bruce', *Index on Censorship* 6, pp. 78–85.

21 Strang, J., Darke, S., Hall, W., Farrell, M. and Ali, R. (1996) 'Heroin overdose: the case for take-home naloxone', *British Medical Journal* 312: 1,435–6.

22 Medicus (1901) 'Heroin overdose' (letter), *British Medical Journal* (26 October): 1,312.

23 Manges, M. (1899) 'The treatment of coughs with heroin', *New York Medical Journal* 68: 768–70.

24 Dreser, H. (1898) 'Ueber die wirkung einiger Derivate des Morphins auf die Athmung' ('On the action of some morphine derivatives on respiration'), *Archiv für Physiologie* 72: 485–521.

25 Higby, G.J. (1986) 'Heroin and medical reasoning: the power of analogy', *New York State Journal of Medicine* 86: 137–41.

26 Brouet, G. (1953) 'The use of heroin in therapeutics', *Bulletin on Narcotics*: 17–18.

27 An amendment to the Harrison Act banned the importation of opium to the United States 'for the purpose of manufacturing heroin' in 1924. However, hospitals were allowed to continue using existing stocks. Jefferson Hospital, Philadelphia, was able to spin out its supplies by judicious prescribing, until finally forced to yield up the little that remained in 1960 as a late response to the Narcotic Control Act. See A.M. Mondzac (1984) 'In defence of the reintroduction of heroin into American medical practice and H.R. 5290 – the Compassionate Pain Relief Act', *New England Journal of Medicine* 311: 533–5.

28 Vaille, C. (1963) 'The use of diamorphine in therapeutics', *Bulletin on Narcotics* 15: 1–5.

29 Trebach, A. (1984) 'Heroin and pain relief', *The Journal*: 5.

30 'Heroin for cancer: a great non-issue of our day', *Lancet* (30 June 1984): 1,449–50.

31 Wolff, P.O. (1956) 'Heroin from the international point of view', *British Journal of Addiction* 53: 51–63.

32 'Symposium on the proposed legislation banning the legal production of heroin in Great Britain', *British Journal of Addiction* 53 (1956): 39–50.

33 Macdonald, A.D. (1956) 'The proposed banning of heroin production', *British Journal of Addiction* 53: 65–8.

34 Subcommittee on Health and the Environment, House of Representatives (1984) *Compassionate Pain Relief Act; Hearings on H.R. 4762*, Washington, D.C.

35 Trebach, A.S. (1982) *The Heroin Solution*, New Haven: Yale University Press.

36 Subcommittee on Health and the Environment, House of Representatives (1980) *Narcotics Abuse and Control*, Washington, D.C.

37 Stoll, S.M. (1985) 'Why not heroin? The controversy surrounding the legalization of heroin for therapeutic purposes', *Journal of Contemporary Health Law and Policy* 1: 173–92.

38 Twycross, R.G. (1974) 'Clinical experience with diamorphine in advanced malignant disease', *International Journal of Clinical Pharmacology* 9: 184–98.
39 Methodist Hospital of Indiana (1976) *A Primer on Brompton's Cocktail*, Indianapolis: Methodist Hospital of Indiana.
40 Twycross, R. (1977) 'Value of cocaine in opiate-containing elixirs', *British Medical Journal* (19 November): 1,348.
41 Twycross, R.G. (1973) 'Euphoriant elixirs', *British Medical Journal* (1 December): 891.
42 Grady, K.M. and Severn, A.M. (1997) *Key Topics in Chronic Pain*, Oxford: Bios Scientific, pp. 50–2.
43 This comes from an anonymous editorial ('Heroin for cancer: a great non-issue of our day', 1984, see note 30 above) but style and content indicate that Twycross was almost certainly the author.
44 International Narcotics Control Board (2000) *Report for 1999*, Vienna: United Nations.

8 *Shots from the drug pub*

The treatment of heroin addiction

The gravity of a disease may be gauged by the number of cures for it. The more cures, the more incurable it is. Judged by this criterion, addiction is a very serious disease indeed.

Dr E.W. Adams[1]

As soon as each had eaten the honeyed fruit of the plant, all thoughts of reporting to us or escaping were banished from his mind. All they now wished for was to stay where they were with the Lotus-eaters, to browse on the lotus, and to forget that they had a home to return to ... . I had to use force to bring them back to the ships, and they wept on the way, but once on board I dragged them under the benches and left them in irons.

Homer, *Odyssey*[2]

Strong treatments

A new treatment regime for heroin addiction has been established recently in Yekaterinburg, Russia. In reaction to the perceived failure of the Sverdlovsk Narcological Hospital, the local anti-drugs programme has been forcibly usurped by Uralmarsh, a syndicate of gangsters, which had previously concentrated successfully on crime. Supply reduction is now implemented energetically by abducting and beating up dealers. Their treatment philosophy is equally straightforward: 'Our concept is that a drug addict is a wild beast, an animal, who cannot be treated with pity.'

They have set up a hotline for relatives, and established a treatment centre in an abandoned rest home twenty miles outside the town. Parents are promised that their children will be kept chained until they are free of drugs. New patients have their hands manacled to radiators above their heads for the first week, except when they eat or relieve themselves. The second week they are allowed short walks. During the third, if all goes well, they are handcuffed only at night. The centre is largely managed by ex-addicts, who often administer violent punishment for non-compliance or attempts to escape.

The programme lasts for about thirty days. Local parents are enthusiastic and queue up to have their addicted children admitted. Many patients are also appreciative. 'There is no other way,' said twenty-four-year-old Dima Gorsky, one of the first to complete the programme. 'The only thing that worked for me is handcuffs. I feel great, better than ever.'[3]

An official version of this system used to prevail in the United States. Between 1927 and 1944 the only authorised treatment for narcotic addiction was within 'drug farms'. Although nominally run by the Public Health Service, they were supervised by the Justice Department and the Federal Bureau of Narcotics, under the ultimate jurisdiction of the Secretary to the Treasury. The institutions established included those in Lexington in Kentucky, Fort Worth in Texas and Spadra in California. In many states these were the only alternative to the workhouse. On admission to drug farms these so-called 'bluegrass' prisoners were bathed, searched, checked for contagious disease and deprived of their civilian clothes. Drugs were generally withdrawn by the 'iron man treatment', in other words abruptly. The regime that followed was organised around physical labour and usually lasted six to nine months. In the words of one commentator,

> the maximum security conditions and cells and bars were familiar to the wardens who transferred thousands of their patients ... the narcotic farms were designed to be and became separate prisons for addicts.[4]

These institutions had closed by the end of the war because the drug menace had abated and also because they were found to be ineffective. Spadra achieved a 'cure rate' of only 15 per cent. Nonetheless, interest in enforced treatment was revived in the early 1960s when drug use began to increase once more. California established a comprehensive system of 'civil commitment' which has remained in force to the present day, and has been copied by New York and several other legislatures. Under this law, addicts can be committed to compulsory care for up to seven years without first being convicted of a criminal offence.[5]

China also favours a robust approach to drug dependence. In 1995 the authorities established over 200 'Centres for the Forcible Termination of Drug Use'. These are supervised by the police and based around hard physical labour. Inmates stay for about six months. They are not allowed to leave, and mail and belongings are regularly inspected. After discharge regular urine tests are taken. Supervision is the responsibility of the family, the work unit and the neighbourhood committee, who are all legally obliged to notify the police if the patient relapses. In theory, getting hold of heroin should be difficult because dealers are likely to suffer public execution. If, nonetheless, former inmates manage to relapse, they are treated as hardened criminals and sent to 'Institutes of Education through Labour'.[6]

It is clear that many people think that forcible treatment is the best option for addiction and indeed sometimes the addicts themselves agree. Many addicts signed up in the 1950s for the Synanon rehabilitation houses founded by Chuck Dederich[7] in the US. Membership involved surrendering all personal rights and initially being treated as a child without any ability to make personal decisions. Slow progress towards normal rights and responsibilities could only be taken after being broken down personally by forceful re-education and structured humiliation. 'Punishments' for wrong thinking included being dressed in nappies and being the target of 'emotional haircuts', in other words abusive criticism from other members of the community. Initially a messianic figure, Dederich gradually became more unbalanced. Towards the end he demanded that inmates of his houses should be sterilised. This tested their loyalty to the utmost, but many followed his directions. It seems they were willing to follow their leader anywhere provided it led them away from the chaotic misery of their former lives.

Are heroin and other drugs of dependency so powerful that addicts really need to be treated like 'wild beasts' or like babies in nappies? It is true that they can lead to dependence and addiction, and that many addicts commit criminal and dangerous acts. But it is also true that many people use these drugs without becoming dependent or addicted and that many people who are addicted do behave responsibly. Nicotine addicts provide an obvious example. This is a very dangerous habit, but it is recognised generally that smokers are only harming themselves, provided they indulge their habit in privacy. There is no call to imprison smokers or to deprive them of their personal rights. It is many years since a Turkish sultan ordered that smokers should have their noses pierced with their pipes, or since a Russian czar decreed that those found in possession of tobacco should be tortured until they named their supplier.[8] Less robust measures have become fashionable, as indeed they have become generally for heroin addiction.

The problem of addiction

Addiction is not the same as physical dependence. Many people are treated for painful conditions with opiates. Often they will become physically dependent and suffer withdrawal symptoms when the drugs are removed. But only a small proportion of these patients becomes addicted to the drug. For the most part they put up with the withdrawal symptoms without much difficulty and do not continue to think about the drug when it is no longer medically needed.

By addiction we mean a specific psychological state in which the drug takes up an overriding importance in the person's life. When they do not have it, they crave for it. They plan their days around ensuring a regular supply. Other personal goals and interests no longer seem important when the supply is threatened. If they manage to stop using the drug for a time, relapse is often followed by a rapid return of the habit at the same intensity as before the period of abstinence. Addiction can also occur to activities unrelated to drugs. People can become addicted to gambling, to computer games, even to housework. Giving up these activities can lead to physical withdrawal symptoms, such as poor sleep and appetite, sweating, palpitations and headaches.

It is becoming clear that similar brain processes underlie all the addictions and that these processes are intimately connected with the mechanisms of learning and habit formation. All organisms need to develop beneficial routines in order to simplify the million decisions that need to be taken each day. 'Habit is the enormous fly-wheel of society.'[9] When children try out a new behaviour, they may find it gives them satisfaction. It either produces an intrinsic pleasure, like eating ice-cream, or leads to enjoyable social interaction, for example the approval of a teacher or a hug from their mother. In either case, the behaviour is 'rewarded' and is more likely to occur in the future.

This simple principle is the foundation of behavioural psychology. Reward leads to learning. By building on simple sequences of actions it is possible to teach complex behaviours. Pigeons can be taught to play ping-pong, monkeys to recognise playing cards. This is not just a psychological process. It also reflects underlying neuro-chemical changes. Rewards are associated with certain chemical events in the brain and these in turn help to establish nerve connections which increase the likelihood of the rewarded behaviour. We share this chemistry with the rest of the animal kingdom. Drugs of abuse are especially good at inducing repetitive behaviour, in particular repeated drug administration, but they do more than reward the activity of drug administration with a pleasant sensation. They actually hijack the chemical reward system itself.

Most drugs of abuse act partly by means of a brain transmitter called dopamine. Opiates cause a general increase in dopamine in the mesolimbic system, the region associated with emotions and feelings. Stimulants such as cocaine and amphetamine prompt a sudden gush of dopamine in a nearby structure, the nucleus accumbens. The same increases are found when behaviour in animals is rewarded with strong reinforcers, such as food or sex. Withdrawal from alcohol, nicotine, opiates and stimulants causes reduced levels of dopamine in the nucleus accumbens. Other brain transmitters are certainly involved in addiction, for example serotonin, GABA, glutamate and neuropeptide Y. But, although the chemistry is complex and still poorly understood, investigators are focusing more and more on mechanisms that are common to the different drugs of addiction and common to processes of both addiction and learning. Drug addiction is seen in this model as 'an aberrant form of learning, mediated by maladaptive recruitment of memory systems'.[10]

Drugs of abuse can therefore impose themselves on our activities and instil in us routines that come to seem as fundamental as those we have acquired from our earliest childhood. Having breakfast in the morning, defecating after breakfast, cleaning our teeth in the evening – these are all behaviours that may have been with us since before we can remember, that in a way seem part of us and would leave a sense of incompletion and unease if they were suddenly forbidden. In the same way, drug use takes on this feeling of interiority, a sense of intrinsically belonging to us. Stopping drug misuse when the habit is acquired leaves not just a vacuum in terms of occupation and entertainment, but an inner vacuum in one's sense of self.

On top of this the system develops tolerance to the drug. Long-term administration of heroin causes quite profound changes in brain chemistry as part of a compensatory drive to regulate brain activity within defined limits. This process of neuro-adaptation reduces the number and sensitivity of opiate receptors, but also alters signalling systems within the cell, leading to a change in the pattern of protein manufacture by the genes. It therefore takes a long time to return to normal when heroin is stopped. Not only is there an immediate withdrawal reaction but there is also a prolonged syndrome, lasting six months or more, during which the patient feels flat in mood, lacking in energy, troubled by cravings and insomnia, and unable to take pleasure in everyday activity.

Heroin addicts therefore have a lot to contend with when they decide to give up the drug. They will undergo an immediate uncomfortable withdrawal reaction and then more than likely a longer period of several months in which they feel below par, generally sleeping poorly and on edge, and lacking the energy and sense of potential gratification to take up new activities. On top of this, they will feel as if something basic to themselves has been taken away. And all this time they will know that they can put everything right by just scoring some heroin again. No wonder that relapse is common. And no wonder that both patients and observers sometimes feel that forcible treatment is the only answer.

Unfortunately it does not work. It would be nice if it did. At least all those people in prison for drug offences could comfort themselves by thinking that they will come out of custody cured of their habit. In fact they almost invariably relapse, even if they have not already managed to continue their drug use in prison.

People are more than just a test tube of chemical reactions. The neuro-chemical learning processes we have described are intimately linked with the higher mental faculties. The process of learning and forgetting is not just a matter of exposure and avoidance of exposure. The intention of the person undergoing the experience is also critical. Just as people passively receiving opiates for pain management do not usually become addicted, so those who have treatment forced upon them do not usually lose their habit.

A contrary argument has been put forward by those who support the Californian system of civil commitment. They argue that as a result of coerced treatment people stay in treatment for longer. The longer that they stay in treatment, the more likely they are to sort out social problems, avoid crime and enjoy better physical health.[11] Their argument is based largely on the results of enforced methadone maintenance programmes. On grounds of common sense one would expect that people who are obliged to take large amounts of methadone every day would be less likely to use much heroin and would thereby avoid some of the dangers of unclean needles and of the criminal activity needed to fund their habit. Even here the evidence is not very strong and has been hard to replicate elsewhere. A similar venture in New York was judged to be a complete failure.[12]

Methadone treatment will be considered later but, when addicts occasionally ask for forceful treatment to cure them of addiction, they are not usually asking to be forced to take methadone for years on end. They are hoping, like some legislators, that a sharp lesson 'will bring them to their senses'. And this definitely does not happen. Even in China, where 'severity and certainty of punishment are the cores of deterrence', underground heroin use is increasing all the time and fears are expressed that 'Centres for the Forcible Termination of Drug Use' are fast becoming 'centres for drug dealing'.[13]

Gentle treatments

Many argue that coercion and confrontation have quite the opposite effect to that which is intended and that by threatening human freedom they increase resistance to change. It is well known that people sometimes pursue their addiction in the face of huge personal costs. A picture in a medical journal recently showed a lady with facial burns. She had severe lung disease caused by smoking but had nonetheless carried on smoking while wearing her oxygen mask, in spite of previous warnings.[14] You may think she was very stupid, but consider Sigmund Freud.[15] In spite of psychoanalysis to stop him smoking, after an operation for mouth cancer he specifically asked that his jaw could be reconstructed in such a way that he would still be able to smoke his cigar. He was in good company. Almost a quarter of patients continue to smoke after heart bypass surgery.[16]

One of the author's patients was admitted to hospital for multiple vein thrombosis as a result of heroin injection. The only vein that doctors could find to insert a drip was the subclavian vein, the big vessel that can be found by inserting a needle below the collar-bone and which runs directly into the main vessels serving the heart. They wondered why the drip kept clotting up. The author had to advise them not to give him painkilling tablets. He was secreting them in his mouth, crushing them up and then at huge risk injecting them straight into the intravenous line. If people on occasions defy imminent death to pursue their addiction, it is unlikely that fear of less severe punishment will bring about a cure.

One way of looking at addiction is to see it as a kind of seesaw. Addicts are aware of the advantages of stopping, but they are also aware of the disadvantages. People only become addicted because the habit serves some useful function. People may use heroin because they enjoy it, because it is an important feature in their social world, because it blots out painful memories or for a hundred other reasons. When they have overindulged or got into trouble, they will become more aware of the advantages of abstinence. As they consider this possibility more seriously the seesaw begins to move down on that side. As that happens, their anxieties about abstinence become more intense. The seesaw begins to rise. Once again they focus on the perils of drug use. The seesaw begins to fall.

This is ambivalence. It lies at the heart of the psychology of addiction. It can be reproduced in animal experiments, in the so-called 'approach/avoidance conflict'. If an animal is confronted at the same time with a feared and an attractive stimulus of equal strength, it can find itself caught indefinitely in a state of suspension. It will move some distance forward, and then some distance back, until it ends up in a state of oscillation round a central point.

Recognising and working with this ambivalence is the guiding principle of 'motivational interviewing', which has recently become perhaps the most widely used form of therapy for addictions. According to its practitioners, confrontation and coercion are the same as putting one's weight on one side of the balance point. The patient is then obliged to press in the other direction to keep some equilibrium. Straight confrontation is therefore counterproductive.[17] Progress is made by recognising that patients spontaneously pass through a 'cycle of change' in their own relationship to their addiction.[18] At times they feel reasonably happy with their habit. At other times they experience some discontent and contemplate change. This may lead them on to take action and, if successful, to achieve abstinence or moderate consumption. Alternatively they may slip back into what therapists call 'pre-contemplation', which is perhaps more accurately called 'untroubled use'. If they manage to control their habit, they will need to maintain the gains made. Or they may relapse and the cycle starts again.

Even without treatment, typical addicts will pass through this cycle on average seven times before achieving successful abstinence. Addicts are always busy dealing with their own addiction. The role of the therapist is to nudge this process forwards, taking careful account of the stage in the cycle that the patient has reached. For example, direct suggestions will be useful as contemplation passes into action. They will generate resistance during 'pre-contemplation'. At this time the task of the therapist is to express understanding; to amplify a sense of discrepancy in the patient's mind between where they are and where they want to be; and to support and strengthen the patient's belief in their own ability to make changes.[19]

Motivational interviewing is at the opposite pole from the Russian handcuff treatment. It is subtle in its respect for complex mental processes and the need to 'roll with them' rather than fight against them. It recently performed very well in a huge American study of alcohol treatment called 'Project Match', by and large doing as well in four sessions as more traditional treatments performed in twelve.[20] It is popular with purchasers of treatment, because brief therapy means cheap therapy. It is widely used to treat heroin addicts.[21] But unfortunately there is little evidence so far to indicate it is effective in treating heroin addiction.

There are many other contenders for the position of best therapy for heroin addiction. 'Relapse prevention' is a behavioural approach that helps people to understand on a day-to-day basis the situations that increase the chance of drug use and to develop strategies and coping mechanisms to avoid or confront these risk occasions.[22] It has long been known that relapse often occurs in response to unsettling or tempting occasions. It has also been recognised that the recovering addict may subconsciously engineer events so that these occasions occur, thus furnishing themselves with a pretext for slipping back into indulgence. Marcel Proust noted this a hundred years ago:

> the morphinomaniac, persuaded that he has been thrown back by some outside event, at the moment when he was just going to shake himself free from his inveterate habit, feels himself to be misunderstood by the doctor who does not attach the same importance to these contingencies, which he sees as mere disguises assumed by the vice which has never ceased to weigh heavily and incurably upon him while he was nursing his dreams of normality and health.[23]

'Relapse prevention' provides a way for the doctor to work with the addict to help him understand the relationship between these contingencies and the underlying 'vice'. It is not just chance that the patient happened to pass a well-known drug dealing spot yesterday. Just because he had an argument with his wife does not mean he had to use heroin. All these events can be controlled, avoided, anticipated or dealt with in some other manner.

'Twelve-step treatment' is the name given to the treatment developed by Alcoholics Anonymous[24] that has extended its scope to take on other addictions through organisations such as Gamblers Anonymous, Cocaine Anonymous and, for heroin addicts, Narcotics Anonymous. This movement has always been more popular in the United States than elsewhere, perhaps because of a traditional sympathy with evangelical Christianity. Affiliation to the movement involves accepting that addiction is a lifelong illness and that abstinence is the only answer. Accepting one's weakness and examining oneself fearlessly as one passes through the twelve steps of treatment enables one to draw strength from 'a Power greater than ourselves' and from colleagues in the movement. The strong support available to those who commit themselves to the movement has helped many people, but it has never had the same impact in heroin addiction as it has had with alcoholism. This may partly be a result of the much smaller percentage of professional people addicted to heroin as opposed to alcohol. The structure provided by regular meetings can provide a lifeline for some people whose lives have become disorganised through drug misuse, but for many chaotic heroin users it remains 'a bridge too far'.

There are many other types of psychotherapy. The advantage of a brief review is that one can make sweeping statements it would take many volumes to defend properly. Faced with a huge variety of therapies, from 'structural family' to 'primal scream', it is time to abridge this chapter by making a disappointing observation. There is no form of psychotherapy at all that has consistently been shown to produce a rate of long-term abstinence from heroin higher than is found with no treatment at all. There are many forms of therapy which have been shown to produce short-term gains. But, in the context of a habit that lasts generally for many years, there is no form of psychotherapy that has been shown to produce any definite impact on the length and severity of a drug user's career.

This negative statement must be placed in context. Until recently most heroin addiction has occurred in deprived neighbourhoods and most of those taking part in treatment surveys come from the same background. Most of the patients' friends take heroin. Most of them have no qualifications and no history of employment. Many have serious histories of childhood abuse and a substantial criminal record. Day-to-day life is crowded with adversity and rich with the type of incident that would push most of us into despair. Routes into other ways of life are few or none. In this context heroin serves a helpful function. It offers pleasure and numbs pain. It gives a focus to a day's activity. The ritual of heroin use also provides social cement and a chance for fellowship. Against this background a few sessions of psychotherapy can seem like shouting in the wind.

But this is not because the drug itself has irresistibly addictive properties. As the more comfortably-off begin to use heroin, no doubt their response to therapy will be as positive as it is in the treatment of other addictions.

Turkey roast – withdrawal from heroin

Medical treatment of heroin addiction merged seamlessly with the treatment of morphinism. The parameters were laid down very early:

'The treatment of the morphia habit is of three kinds: sudden deprivation, gradual deprivation and substitution.'[25] These remain the
mainstays of treatment today. Throughout the twentieth century physicians have introduced many radical treatments, some sensible and
some bizarre, but none have proved reliably efficacious and therefore
each in turn has disappeared. In the next chapter we will discuss treatments based on quite different principles which are likely to emerge
during the next decade. For the moment, however, it must be said that
we have not made a huge amount of progress over the last century. We
are better than we were at alleviating acute withdrawal symptoms. This
is the easy part. However, no medicines have yet proved themselves
capable of meeting the more important challenge of reducing the rate
of relapse.

At the start of the last century doctors thought heroin withdrawal
to be worse than morphine withdrawal, and frequently dangerous.
They observed

> episodes of suffocation, ending frequently in respiratory syncope
> ... . The organism seems to be much more deeply intoxicated ...
> not for four or five months do they regain their weight or begin to
> have undisturbed nights.[26]

Nowadays we would say that the symptoms of morphine and heroin
withdrawal are fairly similar, and that both are rather better than those
found with methadone.

The observed danger of respiratory collapse is odd, even though it
was frequently mentioned at that time. There has been general agreement since then that, however uncomfortable withdrawal may be, it does
not pose any serious risk to health. The only episodes of respiratory
collapse we have seen in the course of many hundreds of detoxifications
occurred when patients took heroin surreptitiously, forgetting they had
partly lost their tolerance. This may well have happened also in the early
clinics without the doctors' knowledge. At the same time many of these
patients suffered from severe tuberculosis and this may perhaps have
explained their sudden deterioration.

The variability of heroin withdrawal symptoms has puzzled doctors.
Some addicts describe it as 'no more rigorous than a nasty dose of
flu'.[27] Others complain more bitterly, for example Rent Boy in Irvine
Welsh's *Trainspotting*:

> A toothache starts tae spread fae ma teeth intae ma jaws and ma
> eye sockets, and aw through ma bones in a miserable, implacable,

debilitating throb. The auld sweats arrive oan cue, and lets no forget the shivers, covering ma back like a thin layer ay autumn frost oan a car roof.[28]

It has long been recognised that symptoms are milder in police custody, where there is no possibility of obtaining drugs,[29] and also that they can be abolished on occasions by the injection of sterile water.[30] These observations have encouraged debate as to whether the symptoms are genuine or 'just psychological'. Dr A.B. Light considered this issue after extensive studies of heroin withdrawal in the 1920s:

> One group holds strongly to the belief that the whole picture is one of hysteria, similar to the hysteria of a child who is deprived of its toy and is promptly seized with an attack of vomiting. Those holding to the other belief insist on somatic changes due to deprivation of the drug.

He inclined to the psychological explanation, observing that similar symptoms of yawning, restlessness and so on were often noted in football players before an important game:

> The players will state they are so weak that they can scarcely move: yet when the whistle starting the game is blown, all fatigue quickly disappears.[30]

This judgement was a little severe. He may have been right that the restlessness experienced in withdrawal is like that felt before a big event. But, when we feel extremely nervous before a speech or an exam, we know that we will soon get relief. The unpleasantness of withdrawal lies in its constant duration over days. Moreover, the positive effect of sterile water does not prove that the discomfort is imaginary. It may be equally effective in severe pain. We now know that the body can mobilise its own endorphins to combat pain over a short period and that placebo medication can stimulate this response. There is no doubt that heroin withdrawal produces an unpleasant physical reaction, although its severity varies from person to person and between different situations. Anybody who has seen the writhing and twitching of patients withdrawn under general anaesthesia will certainly acknowledge that the physical system is undergoing genuine distress.

What A.B. Light was describing were the symptoms of excessive adrenal activity. These occur during extreme excitement, when adrenalin pulses through the blood and gears up the body for immediate action. A major action of heroin and other opiates is to suppress adrenal gland activity by working on their control centre in the brain, the locus coeruleus. When the suppressive action of heroin is removed, the control centre responds by stimulating the adrenal glands excessively. Adrenalin is responsible for many of the uncomfortable symptoms of withdrawal. These include the restlessness, yawning and perspiration which users call 'roasting' or 'rattling'. It also causes the widened pupils, and goose-pimpled flesh which resembles the skin of a plucked turkey. Heroin also reduces bowel movement. Cessation therefore leads to compensatory overactivity and diarrhoea.

Less easy to explain are the 'bone pains' which many find distressing. They are probably due to muscle spasms, but they have given rise to the widespread lay belief that drugs 'get into the bones' and that leaching them out is a painful business. Methadone has got a particular reputation for 'getting into the bones' and, in our experience, patients often give this as a reason for refusing to take it.

Standard early treatments were based on purging the system with laxatives, on sedation and on the use of medicines akin to belladonna.[31] Both purging and belladonna appear strange to the modern observer, as they would tend to exacerbate the symptoms. They were used because they were opposite in action to heroin and would therefore 'stimulate the centres that had been benumbed'.[32] Nowadays we think they are already sufficiently stimulated by the process of withdrawal and therefore look for ways to calm them down. However, a high dose of belladonna had the additional advantage of causing confusion, so the patients may not have noticed.

Some doctors at the time recognised the presence of sympathetic overactivity and regretted that there were no medications that could specifically block this effect. The early 1970s saw the discovery of a new blood-pressure medicine named clonidine.[33] It worked directly on the locus coeruleus and was therefore also useful in heroin withdrawal. But it was also a treatment for hypertension and so sometimes caused alarming falls in blood pressure. A related drug named lofexidine was rejected at the time as a hypertension treatment because it had a weak effect. Later it was rediscovered as a treatment for opiate withdrawal because it had the same effect on the locus coeruleus without causing blood-pressure problems. It is now standard treatment for withdrawal in the UK[34] and will shortly be introduced into the United States. It definitely makes the process of withdrawal much more comfortable.

Other modern methods include slowing down the process by using long-acting opiates such as buprenorphine and laevo-acetyl-methadone (LAAM) or speeding it up by the use of opiate antagonists such as naloxone and naltrexone. We cannot discuss fully the relative advantages of these different approaches. Nor is there space to do justice to all the creative treatments that have passed into history. These include subcutaneous injection of oxygen;[35] replacement of 'nervous system lipids' by various lipid solutions, most commonly one called Narcosan;[36] the production of artificial blisters, followed by injection of blister fluid under the skin;[37] bromide sleep treatment;[38] the injection of sex hormones;[39] electro-convulsive therapy (ECT);[40] and psychosurgery.[41]

The American physician Lawrence Kolb systematically debunked many outlandish treatments some seventy years ago. But credulity does not disappear so easily. The United Nations has been funding the development of a 'miracle' Vietnamese medicine called Heantos, concocted from thirteen local herbs by a traditional healer.[42] A surgeon in St Petersburg is claiming 70 per cent cure rates with a new form of psychosurgery.[43] Meanwhile in Siberia Dr Vladimir Svevchenko has been heating up patients' bodies to the point of hyperthermia in the belief that this 'kills the bad cells, which are causing the physical addiction'.[44] Many patients value 'electro-stimulation',[45] mega-vitamin treatment[46] and acupuncture,[47] even though there is no good evidence that they work better than placebo. But then placebos can be quite effective and at least they are safer than brain surgery.

A dispute that persists is that between gradual and sudden withdrawal. Ultra-rapid detoxification under anaesthesia has recently made a hesitant comeback. In the 1930s 'abrupt withdrawal under hypnosis' was quite popular, using sedatives such as paraldehyde and barbiturates. One contemporary reviewer remarked that these treatments 'do not appear to have attracted many disciples, and indeed the inconveniences of the method (to say nothing of the possible risks) are obvious'.[48] Modern champions[49] claim that it reduces distress, helps those who have failed standard techniques and makes withdrawal attractive to those who would otherwise be frightened off. The contrary view is that the increased risks involved in an anaesthetic cannot be justified:

> While some see these techniques as a 'magic bullet', a miracle breakthrough, others see them as a shameless exploitation of the addict and the general public, the use of a technique with potentially serious morbidity and mortality for a condition that while painful is not associated with mortality.[50]

Unfortunately there is no magic bullet. Whether detoxification takes place abruptly or very slowly, relapse rates remain very high. Helping people get off heroin is not usually a problem. Techniques of detoxification are already sophisticated and usually successful. Until, however, there are better ways of helping people remain abstinent after detoxification, the increased risks associated with rapid detoxification under anaesthesia are probably not justified.

Maintenance care and 'harm reduction'

So what can help in the meantime? As we have argued earlier, many heroin users give up the drug of their own accord. Spontaneous recovery occurs as a result of spiritual experiences, of changes in responsibilities, of new relationships or of a sudden feeling of self-disgust. It usually occurs after many revolutions round the 'cycle of change' and after many short periods of abstinence. At least 5 to 10 per cent manage this every year. The figures are not available to make proper calculations; moreover, they probably change with each new cohort of users and are different in every society. A rough estimate is that the average length of a serious heroin-using career is about fifteen to twenty years. This figure is independent of treatment. There is no evidence to date that any form of treatment makes any difference to length of heroin use. In other words, people give up heroin when they are ready to do so. Events in their lives are much more important in making this decision than anything that occurs in a clinic.

For this reason, the focus has shifted to helping people stay safe and well during the years that they maintain their habit. If they cannot stop using drugs, why not provide them with a safe supply of pharmaceutical opiate? In this way they can be removed from the dangers of the street market and helped to use drugs in a regulated manner. Because their supply is assured, they no longer need to think about drugs all the time. Hopefully the subject will come to seem boring as a topic of thought and they can start to develop other more profitable interests and habits. And, when they are ready to stop using, their health will not have been irrevocably damaged.

This was a common approach during the last century, when chemists and doctors were happy to dispense regular supplies of morphine and laudanum. When heroin became a problem in the United States, a number of clinics were established which dispensed heroin and morphine on this basis. One of the first was that set up by Charles Terry, City Health Officer at Jacksonville, Florida. He also wrote – with Mildred Pellens, his research assistant and later his wife – one of the classic texts on opiate addiction: *The Opium Problem*.[51] In it Terry argued for tolerant and dispassionate research into the addiction, and for medical and social help for opiate addicts rather than legal harassment. Unfortunately, his book only sold 395 copies out of a 2,000 print run and his recommendations were mostly ignored or forgotten until his rediscovery recently as a forerunner of modern treatment methods. His clinic was closed and he later moved to Connecticut where he became an unsuccessful turkey farmer. He finally died while working as a psychiatrist at a small mental hospital in New York State.[52]

The American view of opiate addiction changed radically after the Harrison Act of 1914. Curiously, the Harrison Act was originally very similar to the British Dangerous Drugs Act of 1920; in fact the British Act used the American Act as a model. Both Acts allowed doctors to prescribe opiates in good faith and as part of medical treatment. However, legal interpretation of the Acts turned out to be spectacularly different. In the United States the court was asked to rule on the case of a doctor and a pharmacist who had been supplying morphine to support an addict's habit. Their ruling was clear:

> To call such an order for the use of morphine a physician's prescription would be so plain a perversion of meaning that no discussion of the subject is required.[53]

In Britain, the same question was referred to the Rolleston Committee. They saw things differently: maintenance prescription should be allowed for

> persons for whom, after every effort has been made for the cure of the addiction, the drug cannot be completely withdrawn, either because:- 1) complete withdrawal produces serious symptoms which cannot be satisfactorily treated under the ordinary conditions of private practice; or 2) the patient, while capable of leading a useful and fairly normal life so long as he takes a certain non-progressive quantity, usually small, of the drug of addiction, ceases to be able to do so when the regular allowance is withdrawn.[54]

These two judgments led to a divergence between the two countries. Although later American cases went the other way (for example., *Lindner* v. *US* 1925 and *Boyd* v. *US* 1926), it was too late to save the clinics in Jacksonville, Shreveport and elsewhere which had attempted to treat addicts by maintenance prescription. For the next forty years, the main weapons in the US against opiate misuse were forcible detoxification and legal sanctions. In Britain, the problem was very much smaller. A few physicians continued to prescribe heroin, morphine and cocaine to the small number of addicts who required this treatment. This divergence continued until the mid-1960s.

What changed all this was the discovery of methadone. The Germans in World War II had invented methadone as a synthetic alternative to opiate analgesics, when they lost regular access to the Turkish poppy fields. In 1962 Vincent Dole, a metabolic disease specialist, was asked to take over as Chair of the New York City Health Research Council's Committee on Narcotics while the incumbent went off on sabbatical. As he knew nothing about drug addiction, he enlisted the help of Marie Nyswander. She was a psychiatrist and psychotherapist with extensive experience of addiction, first at Lexington and more recently in charge of a clinic for heroin-addicted jazz musicians.[55] Together they started investigating the effects of opiates on drug users. They discovered that different opiates had different effects. As Nyswander reported,

> With heroin and morphine, the dosage increased irregularly ... and I was writing orders round the clock ... the patients never got dressed, never had any goals other than waiting for the next shot.

In early 1964 came the ice-cream experience. Two patients were switched to methadone and their behaviour changed dramatically. They got up, got dressed and even began going to night school. They reported to her that they had been out in the streets without any problems. 'We saw people scoring for drugs across the street, and we weren't tempted. Instead we went and got an ice-cream cone.'[56]

Dole and Nyswander began to argue strongly for methadone maintenance treatment. Their advocacy came at the right time, because there had been a recent increase in American heroin use. Moreover, the introduction of chlorpromazine as a treatment for schizophrenia had encouraged those who hoped to find medicines that could treat behavioural problems. Dole and Nyswander produced an influential paper in which they showed huge decreases in criminal activity in heroin addicts treated with methadone over the course of a year.[57] By 1970 there were a thousand patients in methadone treatment in New York. Jerome Jaffe, President Nixon's 'drug czar', made methadone maintenance the cornerstone of his national treatment programme. By 1973 there were 80,000 Americans enrolled in methadone programmes.

Not only did Dole and Nyswander see methadone as a way of providing a safe supply of opiate medication. They also came to understand it as a metabolic treatment akin to insulin in diabetes. They reasoned that those who became addicted had some 'persistent neurochemical disturbance'. Through their addiction they had undergone a permanent metabolic change. For this reason they would need lifelong treatment. Because of its long half-life compared to heroin, methadone was able to achieve a pretty steady concentration at the brain's opiate receptors. In this way the brain's function was normalised again, something that did not happen with heroin because the continued ups and downs in the blood concentration of this short-acting drug inevitably led to metabolic instability.[58]

These arguments impressed many British physicians. Following some uninhibited prescribing by a handful of London doctors, the UK system had recently been changed. The treatment of drug addicts had been taken away from GPs and entrusted to newly established specialist clinics. A special Home Office licence was now required to prescribe heroin and cocaine. Specialists were keen to establish their scientific credentials. The new US methadone data were more impressive than anything that had been produced in England. Gradually methadone displaced heroin as the drug of choice for opiate addiction. This process accelerated when an influential London study purported to show that methadone was more effective than heroin.[59]

Although there was a reaction against methadone in the US in the late 1970s when cocaine abuse surpassed heroin as the main drug problem, it has come back into its own with the arrival of AIDS. HIV is spread by sharing injecting equipment. In many of the major world cities, over 60 per cent of drug injectors suffer from HIV infection. There is a clear risk also to the non-drug-using population from this pool of infection. Public health required that as many drug users as possible were induced into treatment and weaned away from the injection of street drugs.

Methadone programmes spread through many areas of the world, for example most of Europe, Australia and many Asian countries. But they continue to be resisted elsewhere, particularly in Russia, China and India. France as usual showed an independent spirit by choosing to base its programme around another opiate: buprenorphine. As buprenorphine is safer in overdose and easier in withdrawal, it is beginning now to win converts in the rest of Europe, Australia and even in the United States.

Along with methadone came the philosophy of 'harm reduction'. It was important not only to provide a substitute for heroin, but also to encourage those who injected to do so in a safe way. This remains controversial. Some countries, for example Holland and the United Kingdom, have been enthusiastic about introducing needle exchange programmes (where old needles can be exchanged for new ones with impunity) and encouraging health workers to teach drug users how to inject safely.

In Germany, Switzerland and Australia special injecting rooms have been established, where users can inject using clean equipment and under professional guidance. For example, nuns are set to run Australia's first legal injecting room in the Kings Cross red light district in Sydney. They expect 50,000 visits a year and will provide clean needles, syringes, showers, a subsidised café, security guards and encouragement to seek help and counselling. 'We've reflected on our traditional Catholic moral teaching,' reported Dr Tina Clifton, chief executive of the Sisters of Charity. 'We believe it supports the sisters' commitment to the preservation of life.' A leading local doctor called it 'one of the most outstanding advances in public health in the drugs debate for twenty years'.[60]

Many countries still remain unconvinced, believing this practice to be immoral or at the very least an encouragement to deviant behaviour. Needle exchange only occurs to a limited extent in the United States and receives no backing from federal funds.[61] Even 'bleach and teach' programmes have been resisted. These are schemes whereby information about safe needle use is propagated, along with instructions on how to sterilise equipment with household bleach. Some of the most vociferous opponents of these schemes have been the community leaders in ethnic strongholds such as Harlem, who see them as demeaning and corrupting to their people.[62]

Extensive reviews have established beyond doubt that methadone treatment is very effective in preserving health, reducing crime, reducing the spread of infection and lessening overdose death. It is calculated that heroin – injecting addicts have a mortality rate sixteen times higher than their non-injecting peers. On methadone programmes this increase in mortality reduces to only double. But they have also established that methadone treatment is not a 'cure'. Many of those who remain in treatment continue to use heroin, albeit at much reduced doses. Those who leave treatment tend to relapse. Treatment should therefore be for as long as it is required.[63]

There is a tendency, particularly in Europe and Australia, for methadone to be seen not as a metabolic treatment for heroin addiction, but as 'a guaranteed supply of legal pharmaceutical opioid leading to a range of secondary benefits as the activity of illicit drug taking is reduced or stopped'.[64] Opiates themselves are not dangerous. The harm is caused by the illegal and unhygienic practices associated with undercover use. The idea of treatment is to provide a safe alternative, like nicotine patches for smokers but over a longer period of time. But if this is the case, why not give them heroin? Heroin is, after all, their drug of addiction and indeed quite a high number of heroin users dislike methadone. In the words of one consumer, 'I hate the way it looks, I hate the way it tastes and if it made a sound, I'm sure I would hate that too.'[65] Many dislike the feeling of 'being wrapped in cotton wool' that it can produce. Many also find that withdrawal symptoms are worse when they try to stop than when they come off heroin. For these reasons, a sizeable number of drug users are unwilling to come into treatment when all that is on offer is methadone.

In fact heroin prescription is currently under investigation in Switzerland, Holland and Germany as an alternative to methadone. The Swiss have shown that it is feasible to maintain addicts on injectable heroin, on the basis that they attend three times a day at an injecting room for their injections. A number of addicts who had not responded well to methadone treatment have shown reductions in criminal activity and improvements in health.[66] The Dutch are investigating smokable as well as injected heroin. They dispense it by means of tablets that are heated on electric rings. The tablets also contain caffeine to enhance pulmonary absorption. A handful of British doctors have continued to prescribe heroin under Home Office licence and are aware how beneficial it can be for some patients.

What has become clear through this experience is that much higher doses of heroin are needed to produce mental stability than was previously thought. The Swiss use on average 600 mg a day, whereas the British study referred to above used only 100 mg a day. Had Marie Nyswander treated her patients with higher doses of heroin, perhaps the superior advantages of methadone would not have impressed her so strongly.

Conclusion

All this means that for many people the treatment of heroin addiction consists of keeping them safe by providing them with a regular supply of the drug of their choice, along with clean needles and information about safe consumption. 'For God's sake, just give them the drugs,' as William Burroughs is reported to have said when his typewriter was stolen. Recovery will occur when people are ready for it, but may perhaps be encouraged by low-key, finely tuned intermittent counselling.

Described in this way treatment appears rather feeble. The public is not impressed, and cannot understand why patients receive a daily dole of medication without ever getting over their addiction. Some observers suspect a hidden agenda. 'Methadone is not a treatment, it is a method of social control.'[67] Many would agree with the opinion of the original US anti-drugs boss, Harry Anslinger, in relation to the first drug clinics in the United States:

> It is interesting to note that most of the advocates of this system do not even go so far as to advocate a cure. It is simply set forth as a plan whereby the addict maintains his old habit and invariably returns to the clinic where a fresh supply is administered or given to him for a small sum, and the victim again set at large to contaminate others to his ranks; this procedure to be continued indefinitely.[68]

But there is another way of looking at it. If you want to drink alcohol, you buy it in a shop. If you prefer to use opiates, there is no legal way you can obtain them except by attending a treatment programme. If you ask for treatment for alcohol addiction, it is because you are in serious trouble and want to stop buying alcohol. If you attend a heroin treatment programme, it may be that you want to go on taking opiates but no longer have the stomach for breaking the law. Of course you will say you want to 'come off' and you will tell journalists that you haven't been given a chance to get clean. But if you really want to come off heroin, you will do what a small proportion of your mates do every year. They just stop using it.

Until this happens it is right that opiate users should have some legal access to a supply of uncontaminated drugs. When they really want to stop then all necessary help should be at hand, whether medical, social or psychological. But often when they are ready they won't need this extra help. This has been well summarised by Griffith Edwards, an eminent British addiction specialist:

> All recovery is 'natural recovery', with treatment conceived as at best simply the skilful business of nudging and supporting self-determined change … . Perhaps some of the crasser therapeutic approaches which have in the past sought to impose cure on their

patients have in fact been 'unnatural' in their philosophies and fragile outcomes.[69]

There is another more important reason why attracting and retaining people in treatment is beneficial. Anslinger was probably wrong in claiming that 'the victim contaminates others to his ranks' when receiving a prescribed supply of opiates. Thirty years ago Patrick Hughes and his colleagues in Chicago showed just how to snuff out a heroin epidemic:

> Our approach for intervening in heroin spread is based upon established public health principles used to halt epidemics of certain contagious diseases, namely, early identification of new outbreaks and early involvement of all diseased persons in treatment to prevent them from spreading the disorder to others.[70]

When they had identified one heroin user, they interviewed him to find out the names of his using friends, and then recruited his help to find and entice them into treatment. In this manner they tracked their way back down the local networks. By involving all local users at an early stage in the spread of the habit, they frustrated the development of local drug markets. They also found that users in treatment are no longer glamorous and therefore no longer form role models for their peers. There is a world of difference between the 'righteous dope fiend' and the rather sad figure queuing up for methadone. Streetwise youth might want to copy the former, but definitely not the latter. Unfortunately, Hughes' work has largely been forgotten, but we believe that now is the right time for a revival. It may be expensive on resources, but it will definitely be cheaper than dealing with a cohort of end-stage users with terminal AIDS and hepatitis. And it could prevent a mountain of human suffering.

It is therefore sensible to provide access to clean opiates while waiting for the urge towards recovery. And during this time it is best if the doctor does not cut back on the dose of prescription too radically, or they may fall victim to the 'curse of Crowley'. It is reported that Dr William Brown, physician of the English magician Aleister Crowley, systematically reduced his dose of prescribed heroin and stopped it altogether against Crowley's protests in September 1947. On 1 December Crowley died; the very next day Brown was found dead in his bath in his Mayfair apartment. The coroner recorded natural causes for his death, but Crowley's many acolytes concluded it was no such thing. It was the result of his curse on the perpetrator of what Griffith Edwards might have called a 'crass therapeutic approach'.[71]

Notes

1 Adams, E.W. (1937) *Drug Addiction*, Oxford: Oxford University Press, p. 126.
2 In Book IX of the *Odyssey*, stormy winds throw Odysseus and his crew ashore in the land of the Lotus-eaters. This is an early example of forceful treatment of drug abuse, successful because the addicts were thereby permanently removed from their drugs.
3 Slackman, Michael (2000) 'Hard Drugs, Hard Cure', *Newsday* (3 January): 8.
4 Musto, D.F. (1999) *The American Disease: Origins of Narcotic Control*, New York: Oxford University Press, p. 206.
5 Bean, Philip (2000) 'Pressure pays', *Findings* 2: 4–7.
6 Liu, Weizheng and Situ, Yingyi (1996) 'China. The causes, control and treatment of illegal drugs', *Crime and Justice International* 12: 5ff.
7 White, William L. (1998) *Slaying the Dragon. The History of Addiction Treatment and Recovery in America*, Bloomington: Chestnut Health Systems.
8 Working Party of the Royal Colleges of Psychiatrists and Physicians (2000) *Drugs Choices and Dilemmas*, London: Gaskell, p. 29.
9 James, William (1890) *The Principles of Psychology*, New York: Henry Holt, Ch. 4.
10 Robbins, T.W. and Everitt, B.J. (1999) 'Drug addiction: bad habits add up', *Nature* 398: 567–70.
11 Anglin, M.D., Prendergast, M. and Farabee, D. (1998) *The effectiveness of coerced treatment for drug-abusing offenders*, Washington, D.C.: Office of National Drug Control Policy.
12 Inciardi, J.A. (1988) 'Compulsory treatment in New York: a brief narrative history of misjudgement, mismanagement and misrepresentation', *Journal of Drug Issues* 28: 547–60.
13 Liu and Situ (1996).
14 Gujral, J.S. Minerva (1991) *British Medical Journal* 303 (26 October): 1,080.
15 Jones, Ernest (1953) *The Life and Work of Sigmund Freud*, New York: Basic Books. Freud's lifelong struggle with tobacco is summarised in E.M. Brecher (1972) *The Consumers Union Report on Licit and Illicit Drugs*, Boston: Little Brown.
16 Taira, D.A. *et al.* (2000) 'Impact of smoking on health-related quality of life after percutaneous coronary revascularisation', *Circulation* 102: 1,369–74.
17 Miller, W. and Rollnick, S. (eds) (1991) *Motivational Interviewing*, New York: Guilford.
18 Prochaska, J.O. and DiClemente, C.C. (1982) 'Transtheoretical therapy: toward a more integrative model of change', *Psychotherapy: theory, research and practice* 192: 76–288.
19 Miller and Rollnick (1991).
20 Cisler, R., Holder, H. and Longabaugh, R. (1998) 'Actual and estimated replication costs for alcohol treatment modalities: case study from Project Match', *Journal of Studies on Alcohol* 59: 503–12.
21 Saunders, B., Wilkinson, C. and Allsop, S. (1991) 'Motivational interviewing with heroin users attending a methadone clinic', in W.R. Miller

and S.R. Rollnick (eds) *Motivational Interviewing*, New York: Guilford, pp. 279–92.

22 Marlatt, G.A. and Gordon, J.R. (1985) *Relapse Prevention*, New York: Guilford.

23 Proust, Marcel (1960) *Swann's Way*, trans. C.K. Scott Moncrieff, London: Chatto & Windus, part 2, p.125.

24 Kurtz, E. (1979) *Not God: A History of Alcoholics Anonymous*, Centre City: Hazelden.

25 Kane, H.H. (1880) *The Hypodermic Injection of Morphia*, New York: Charles Bermingham, p. 288.

26 Duhem, P. (1907) 'L'héroïne et les héroïnomanes' ('Heroin and heroin addicts'), *Progrès Medicale* 23: 113–17, quoted in *British Medical Journal*, Epitome of Current Medical Literature (June 1st 1907), p. 87.

27 Marlowe, Ann (1999) *How to stop time. Heroin from A to Z*, London: Virago Press, p. 228.

28 Welsh, Irvine (1999) *Trainspotting*, London: Vintage, p. 16.

29 See, for example, W.H. Wilcox (1923) 'Norman Kerr Memorial Lecture on Drug Addiction', *British Medical Journal* (1 December): 1,013–18.

30 Light, A.B. and Torrance, E.G. (1929) 'The effects of abrupt withdrawal followed by readministration of morphine in human addicts', *Archives of Internal Medicine* 44: 1–16.

31 See C.E. Terry and M. Pellens (1928) *The Opium Problem*, Montclair: Patterson Smith, pp. 517–628, for an extensive review.

32 Pettey, G.E. (1913) *The Narcotic Drug Diseases and Allied Ailments*, Tennessee: J.A. Davis, quoted in Terry and Pellens (1928).

33 Pettinger, W.A. (1973) 'Clonidine, a new antihypertensive drug', *New England Journal of Medicine* 293: 1,179–80.

34 See, for example, T. Carnwath and J. Hardman (1998) 'Randomised double-blind comparison of lofexidine and clonidine in the out-patient treatment of opiate withdrawal', *Drug and Alcohol Dependence* 50: 251–4.

35 Bogolow, T.M. (1925) 'Die heilung von Narkomanen durch subkutane Zufuhr von Sauerstoff' ('The treatment of drug addicts by subcutaneous injection of oxygen'), *Moscow Medical Journal*, quoted in Terry and Pellens (1928).

36 Lambert, A. and Tilney, F. (1926) 'The treatment of narcotic addiction by Narcosan', *New York Medical Journal* 124: 764.

37 This is Modinos Autogenous Serum Therapy, based on the idea that opiate addiction was a result of specific antibody development. It achieved quite wide popularity. See P. Modinos (1929) 'La guérison des toxicomanes' ('Curing drug addicts'), *Bulletin de l'Acadamie Medicale de Paris* 102: 83.

38 See H.D. Kleber and C.E. Riordan (1982) 'The treatment of narcotic withdrawal: a historical review', *Journal of Clinical Psychiatry* 43: 30–4. They remark that although there were two deaths among the ten patients so treated, proponents of the treatment still advocated its use in 'well-selected cases'. This paper provides a good review of other treatments not mentioned by ourselves.

39 Luthe, E. and Schmidt, E. (1931) 'Morphiumentziehungsbehandlung mit Anermon und Gynormon' ('Treatment of morphine withdrawal with Anermon and Gynormon'), *Medizine Klinische* 27: 1,038, described along with other hormone therapies in Adams (1937).

40 Thigpen, F.B., Thigpen, C.H. and Cleckley, H.M. (1953) 'Use of electro-convulsive therapy in morphine, meperidine and related alkaloid addictions', *Archives of Neurology and Psychiatry* 70: 452–8.

41 Knight, G. (1969) 'Chronic depression and drug addiction treated by stereotactic surgery', *Nursing Times* 65 (8 May), pp, 583–86.

42 Larimer, T. (1997) 'Laboratory drug wars', *Time* 150 (22 December) 35–8.

43 Fleming, P., Bradbeer, T. and Green, A. (2001) 'Substance misuse problems in Russia. A perspective from St Petersburg', *Psychiatric Bulletin* 25: 27–8.

44 Thomas, Ian (2000) 'This man is being boiled alive to cure his addiction', *Daily Mirror* (23 November): 11.

45 This is a form of acupuncture involving electric stimulation. Sometimes called the 'Black Box' it became popular after the successful treatment of musician Eric Clapton. See M.A. Flowerdew (1998) *General Introduction to Electrostimulation Techniques and the Treatment of Heroin Withdrawal Symptoms*, Liverpool: Drug Free.

46 Libby, A.F. and Stone, I. (1977) 'The hypoascorbemia-kwashiorkor approach to drug addiction therapy: a pilot study', *Journal of Orthomolecular Psychiatry* 6, 4: 300–8. This treatment is based on the notion that drug addiction is due to defective vitamin metabolism and can be corrected by massive doses of vitamins.

47 See G. Ter Riet, J. Kleijnen and P. Knipschild (1990) 'A meta-analysis of studies into the effect of acupuncture on addiction', *British Journal of General Practice* 40: 379–82.

48 Adams (1937), p. 131.

49 Brewer, C. (1997) 'Ultra-rapid antagonist precipitated opiate detoxification under general anaesthesia or sedation', *Addiction Biology* 2: 291–302.

50 Kleber, H.D. (1998) 'Ultra-rapid opiate detoxification', *Addiction* 93: 1,629–33.

51 Terry and Pellens (1928).

52 Kalant, H. (2000) 'Classic texts revisited: *The Opium Problem* by C. Terry & M. Pellens', *Addiction* 95, 101: 585–7.

53 Musto (1999), p. 132.

54 Ministry of Health (1926) *Drug Addiction: Report of the Departmental Committee on Morphine and Heroin Addiction*, London: HMSO.

55 Winick, C. and Nyswander, M. (1961) 'Psychotherapy of successful musicians who are drug addicts', *American Journal of Orthopsychiatry* 31: 622–36.

56 Courtwright, D.T. (1997) 'The prepared mind: Marie Nyswander, methadone maintenance and the metabolic theory of addiction', *Addiction* 92: 257–265.

57 Dole, V.P. and Nyswander, M.E.A. (1965) 'Medical treatment for diacetyl-morphine (heroin) addiction', *Journal of the American Medical Association* 193: 646–50.

58 Dole, V.P. and Nyswander, M.E. (1967) 'Heroin addiction – a metabolic disease', *Archives of Internal Medicine* 120: 19–24.

59 Hartnoll, R.L. *et al.* (1980) 'Evaluation of heroin maintenance in controlled trial', *Archives of General Psychiatry* 378: 877–84.

60 Zinn, S. (1999) 'Nuns to run first heroin injecting room', *British Medical Journal* 319 (14 August): 400.

61 For the official negative view of needle exchange in the US, see Office of National Drug Control Policy (1992) *Needle exchange programs: are they effective?*, ONDCP Bulletin No. 7 (July).

62 Lambert, B. (1988) 'The free-needle programme is under way and under fire', *New York Times* (13 November).

63 Hall, W., Ward, J. and Mattick, R.P. (1998) *Methadone maintenance treatment and other replacement therapies*, Amsterdam: Harwood Academic Publishers.

64 Seivewright, N. (2000) *Community treatment of drug misuse: more than methadone*, Cambridge: Cambridge University Press, p. 23.

65 Newcombe, R. (1998) '*Drug users' views of methadone*', paper presented at Society for the Study of Addictions Methadone Conference, Manchester Metropolitan University.

66 Uchtenhagen, A., Dobler-Mikola, A., Steffen, T., Gutzwiller, F., Blattler, R. and Pfeifer, S. (1999) *Prescription of Narcotics for Heroin Addicts. Main results of the Swiss National Cohort Study*, Basle: Karger.

67 Braid, Mary (2000) 'Methadone – cure or con?', *The Independent: Review* (19 July): 1.

68 Anslinger, H.J. and Tompkins, W.F. (1981) *The Traffic in Narcotics*, New York: Arno Press.

69 Edwards, G. (2000) 'Editorial note: natural recovery is the only recovery', *Addiction* 57: 47.

70 Hughes, P.H. and Crawford, G.A. (1972) 'A contagious disease model for researching and intervening in heroin epidemics', *Archives of General Psychiatry* 27: 149–55.

71 Booth, M. (2000) *A Magick Life*, London: Hodder & Stoughton.

9 *Beyond the needle*
Heroin use in the future

A regime – like that used for alcohol, tobacco and legal pharmaceuticals – which involves legal controls on importation, manufacture, wholesale and retail supply, with rules about hours of supply and ages of those who can buy, with duty and tax extracted at each level and with health and safety controls to ensure standard strengths and remove impurities would at least stand a chance of being effective. It would bring a very substantial business within the law.

Francis Wilkinson, former Chief Constable of Gwent, Wales[1]

I find no merit in the legalisers' case. The simple fact is that drug use is wrong ... . Imagine if in the darkest days of 1940, Winston Churchill had rallied the West by saying 'this war looks hopeless, and besides it will cost too much. Hitler can't be that bad. Let's surrender and see what happens.'

William J. Bennett, former American drug czar[2]

We have attempted to provide a bird's-eye view of how heroin use developed over the last century. Heroin has not been suppressed but has become an unavoidable feature of modern life. Changes have been rapid, but we believe this century will produce much greater changes. New technology will make heroin use more acceptable to middle-class users. This is a process which is already starting to happen, as taboos against other drugs gradually crumble. It will become increasingly clear that the 'war on drugs' is a failure, although this will not stop some last frantic efforts. Mounting concern about international gangsterism and corruption will press governments to take action, eventually to take control of the drug trade themselves.

We believe that heroin use will inevitably be legalised at some point in the future. More controversially, we predict that this will happen quite soon and the first steps will probably take place within the next ten years, with European countries taking the lead. The United

Kingdom is home to the largest drug market in Europe. For that reason it may well move more quickly down this path than other countries which at present have more liberal regimes, such as Holland and Portugal. It would be just if the country that gave heroin to the world were the one that first launched itself with enthusiasm on this hazardous journey. In this chapter we consider how this process might develop and what effects it will have on society.

New techniques for drug use

We have seen how the invention of new techniques revolutionised heroin use, most notably intravenous injection and chasing the dragon. The latter was particularly important because it made heroin use acceptable to people who would have balked at the idea of syringes and tourniquets. Technology does not stand still, nor does drug use. Methods of medical drug administration are evolving at great speed and it would be surprising if, in time, new techniques were not adopted by recreational users. Many of these may well appeal to middle-class users and will thereby hasten the march of heroin out of the sink estates and into the leafy suburbs.

One example is the Powderject system.[3] This can deliver powdered medications directly through the skin without leaving any injection mark. It looks like a conventional syringe but it is tipped with a tiny nozzle rather than a needle. It contains a small gas canister filled with high-pressure helium. A drug cassette is inserted, which contains the powdered drug sandwiched between two plastic membranes. Pressing the trigger allows gas to be released at a designated pressure. The gas ruptures the plastic membranes and forms a shock wave which travels down the nozzle at 600 to 900 metres per second dragging the powdered drug behind it. At this speed the particles painlessly penetrate the skin while the gas is collected back into a silencer. Manipulating the gas pressure accurately calibrates the depth of penetration. If aimed at the precise depth of the skin's blood supply it will be absorbed directly into the bloodstream.

At present this is mostly used for administrating vaccines, but insulin injection for diabetics is another likely use. We spoke to the manufacturers about its potential for drug addicts. They admitted that cocaine or heroin could be used in the system, but someone would have to powder them very finely and then pre-pack them into the special Powderject capsules. For the moment this technology is confined to their factory. However, it is not terribly complicated and it may not be long before rogue operators learn the necessary skills, given the huge financial potential and the growing technological sophistication of suppliers. A more serious problem is that the maximum payload is in the region of 3 mg, which is insufficient to support a serious heroin habit. It is, however, quite adequate for the more potent synthetic opioids such as fentanyl and buprenorphine.

Probably closer to adoption on the street is the Smart Needle system developed by the Peripheral Systems Group in Houston. At present it is undergoing trial in renal dialysis units where patients need multiple intravenous transfusions. Their problem is similar to that of intravenous drug addicts: it becomes increasingly difficult to find usable veins. The smart needle employs sound waves to home in on its target. It harnesses the Doppler effect to detect changes in sound frequency as blood flows through a vein. As the operator moves the needle across the skin the hum becomes louder as he approaches a viable vein.

With this feedback, injectors achieve a near 100 per cent success rate in making clean injections. There is no doubt that this would be very useful for regular heroin injectors and would probably improve their health. And because it is also an elegant electronic gadget it could appeal to a generation fond of mobile phones, PlayStations and personal organisers.[4]

Many new drug delivery systems are designed to produce a steady blood level of drug. Drug users prefer sudden bursts of drug since the 'hit' derives from the sudden change in blood level. Treatment agencies aim for a steadier level, so that patients can avoid not only withdrawal symptoms but also the recurrent hit that keeps them locked into their habit. Doctors view a steady level of prescribed opiate as a halfway house that will allow users time to adjust to life away from their drug-using friends and prepare them for eventual detoxification and abstinence. Methadone is therefore often the drug of choice, because its long half-life allows a steady level in the blood with a once-daily dosage.

Doctors may see the advantage of drug-impregnated skin patches. These foil-backed, adhesive patches set up a tiny electric current that draws the drug out of the patch and into the skin. Fentanyl skin patches are already widely used for the treatment of severe pain and doctors could, in theory, use them for maintaining heroin addicts. In view of anxiety about clinic patients selling on their methadone, doctors might also like the idea of 'bioerodible implants'. These implants work somewhat like the solid air fresheners that gradually release fragrance as they evaporate. A single implant could easily contain a month's supply of fentanyl and be inserted under the skin with a scalpel nick and a stitch.

A new development may make these implants more attractive to drug users. 'Patient-activated' implants respond to ultrasound pulses or magnetic fields. In theory an addict could insert such an implant once a month. They would carry an ultrasound pulser, which could be a device like a wristwatch: whenever they wanted a hit they would just press the button. They would then have all the delights of regular intoxication without the hassle of scoring every day, evading the police, acquiring a hundred needles and syringes a month, and having to search their arms and legs for remotely viable veins. A scalpel nick each month may seem like a good bargain. Ultrasound pulsers can also activate skin patches.

Snorting is how addicts in the US originally used heroin. It is suitable for high-grade diamorphine hydrochloride. It does not occur much in Europe because less concentrated diamorphine base is available on the market and there is not much uptake into the system when this is snorted. There are, however, many recreational drug users who have become experienced in snorting through use of cocaine powder. If heroin could be snorted efficiently it might cause a large expansion of use in this group, particularly as heroin is generally considered a very good drug for easing the comedown after a cocaine high.

New techniques have improved the efficiency of nasal absorption. Insulin can now be administered through the nose. The trick that makes this system work is combining aerosol droplets of insulin with a chemical 'permeation enhancer' that momentarily opens the junctions between nasal cells. Insulin levels in the blood peak about fifteen minutes after administration, closely mimicking the body's normal insulin response to a meal. Nasal delivery systems are currently available for anti-allergy and other medicines. An aerosol combined with a 'permeation enhancer' would be an extremely efficient way of delivering heroin. It would also click with the professional lifestyle. The successful stockbroker could use an aerosol with discretion, but would quickly lose clients if seen fiddling about with syringes and spoons.[5]

Is heroin becoming respectable in Britain?

None of these techniques are close to hitting the streets, but it does not take a crystal ball to foresee them affecting drug misuse over the next twenty years. It is likely that they will assist the move upmarket that we have already described. In the UK heroin is being packaged now in cheap £5 to £10 wraps, whereas before £20 wraps were the normal fare. This implies that the modern customer is the casual user, not just the addict with a heavy habit.

Heroin is now appearing in towns very different from the deprived inner cities. A night out in Macclesfield or Leamington Spa may well take in a little heroin alongside the drinks and cocaine. Recent research has shown that in smaller British cities and towns between five and twenty percent of 15 year olds had been offered heroin, while a quarter said they could easily get the drug.

> It is patently clear from the audit that small cities and towns of all sizes are currently the sites for new outbreaks…. the audit also hinted at wider social dispersal. Numerous respondents suggested that, whilst heroin uptake was still centred in the town's poorest populations, there was also uptake amongst more affluent young people.[6]

The authors point out that this process is similar to that which is already occurring in the United States. All of this is part of a major shift in attitudes to drug use, particularly in the UK which has become the largest consumer market for illicit drugs in Europe.

> Users no longer view drugs as forbidden fruit but instead as tools to maximise the hedonistic pleasure from leisure activities or to perform better at work. This utilitarian mindset is leading users to design their own pharmacopoeia, using one substance to alleviate the adverse effects of another or on the contrary to boost the effects that are perceived as positive. This logic entails the blurring of lines between licit and illicit substances and 'soft' and 'hard' drugs.[7]

Events at a recent Conservative Party conference clearly illustrated this seismic shift in attitudes. Shadow Home Minister Ann Widdecombe hoped for ready applause from the law-and-order constituency when she demanded zero tolerance for cannabis use, and called for spot searches and fixed penalty fines for possession. In fact she stirred up a storm of protest and only narrowly avoided resignation. The Police Superintendents' Association dubbed it unworkable. Shadow cabinet colleagues queued up to embarrass her by confessing to juvenile cannabis use and even to finding it enjoyable. Party supporters in the stockbroker belt foresaw with horror the call to the local nick to bail out their Gavins and Jessicas. Widdecombe's proposal may partly have been aimed at Home Secretary Jack Straw, whose teenage son had been cautioned for cannabis possession only a few months before. But if so it backfired spectacularly. Young William Straw received widespread public sympathy, whereas Widdecombe faced a flood of criticism and was forced into a shamefaced retraction.[8]

But in theory cannabis use is still a crime; indeed it still leads to more prosecutions a year than any other drug. Liberal Party leader Charles Kennedy commented that Widdecombe 'had performed a public service in the past few days by showing how far public attitudes have changed'. He said he did not regard the shadow cabinet members or other recreational users of cannabis as criminals. Asked if he believed the drug should be decriminalised, he answered: 'Yes'.[8]

In terms of British politics, it is remarkable that the Liberal Party leader should thus express agreement with the *Daily Telegraph*, the most right-wing and conservative of British papers. An editorial earlier in the year had proposed that cannabis should be legalised for an experimental period:

> Given that we live in an age in which the drugs of the world have found their way to our shores, surely the truly conservative answer to the problem is to find ways of acclimatising drugs to bourgeois society rather than yelling vainly into the wind ... .
> We do not pretend that this would lead to an end, or even a diminution, of the horrors of addiction. These, after all, are appallingly present with legal alcohol. But we do think that it would start to take power away from criminals, restore a respect for the law, and encourage the drug-affected generations to grow up.[9]

These shifts in attitude are highly significant. Fifty years ago the British considered cannabis as exotic and highly dangerous. A contemporary writer provided a lurid account of a group of Soho jazz musicians called the Vipers, who had 'handed over their souls to marijuana and orgies. The public must know that once they have tasted the vile stuff only a miracle can save them.'[10] Now shadow cabinet ministers approve its use with the support of the *Daily Telegraph*. Fifty years is a short time in the life of a drug. Over that time the British have assimilated spaghetti, yoghurt and Thai curries. Perhaps cannabis is not such a big challenge in comparison, and perhaps the same applies to other drugs as well.

One purpose of this book is to move away from the skirmishes of the present and take a longer-term look at drug history. From this viewpoint it is clear that the same shift of attitude is beginning to occur with cocaine and heroin as has occurred with cannabis, and that it will not be long before the *Daily Telegraph* calls for the legalisation of these drugs as well. All the arguments used in their editorial to justify cannabis legalisation could equally have been applied to heroin.

Not long ago an enterprising journalist trawled through the toilets of the House of Commons and the House of Lords taking samples from flat surfaces. Many samples contained cocaine. The conclusion was inescapable: cocaine snorting occurred even within the hallowed halls of Westminster. Commented Labour MP Paul Flynn:

> At least the myth has been destroyed that if people start out on a soft drug, they end up on heroin. That they end up on the Tory front benches is not an enviable fate, but it is not quite as bad as lying in a gutter with a needle sticking out of you.[11]

This comment is illuminating. As cocaine use spreads through the bars and clubs frequented by journalists and policy-makers, they find it increasingly hard to see cocaine use *per se* as a crime, or even to consider cocaine a 'hard drug'. Heroin remains a fate worse than death, worse even than becoming a Tory minister. But the battleground is shifting. The line between acceptable and unacceptable drugs is moving away from that between legal and illegal. Once it starts moving, who knows where it will stop? These lines can remain stable for decades, but once they start moving they move quickly.

It is a general rule of drug use that *my drug* is an enjoyable recreation and social stimulus, whereas *your drug* is a destructive evil. This is based on custom rather than reason, as is illustrated by alcohol and opium. Alcohol use remains a crime in many countries, but in others it is a key element in social and personal life. Those countries that ban it do so with good logic. It is a potent cause of violent crime, domestic violence, broken homes, car crashes and industrial accidents. It imposes huge costs on industry and the health service. But many countries that ban alcohol had until recent times a long history of sanctioned opium use. One reason for not banning opium in India under the British Raj was the fear that it would be replaced by alcohol. In 1893 a hundred doctors practising in India unanimously agreed 'that the effects of alcohol were far worse than those of opium and that prohibiting opium's use would lead to a rise in alcohol consumption in India'.[12] Nonetheless, most of those who drink alcohol in the UK today consider opium to be a very dangerous drug.

Alcohol, tobacco, coffee and tea have long been permitted drugs among the British ruling classes. These were *my drugs*. Cocaine, cannabis and heroin were taken by the deprived and marginalised, and were therefore seen as dangerous and unhealthy. They were *your drugs. My drugs* were held to be unarguably better than *your drugs,* even though 200,000 people die every year in the UK from the effects of alcohol and tobacco but only about 2,000 from using illicit drugs.

People tend to deal with uncomfortable facts about *my drugs* by distinguishing between sensible and foolish use. This tradition is an old one. King James I pointed out the difference between 'persons of good calling and quality' who took tobacco as 'a physic to preserve their health' and a 'number of riotous and disordered persons of mean and base condition' who spent their time and money on tobacco 'not caring at what price they buy their drug'.[13] Indeed the distinction is justified. Decades of alcohol research have shown conclusively that the higher your social class, the more likely you are to drink frequently, but the less likely you are to drink abusively. And moreover if you do slip up and require treatment, you are much more likely to respond positively to it.[14] The same is true for nicotine.[15]

The attitude to *your drugs* is much less generous. They are seen as being instantly addictive and inevitably leading to ruin and destruction. But the line between *my drugs* and *your drugs* is shifting. As cannabis use becomes more common in privileged circles, influential people are starting to realise that destructive use is not inevitable. People can in truth become addicted to cannabis and cause themselves serious illness, but the great majority of users partake with restraint and pleasure. Cocaine use is probably beginning to move in the same direction. Most young people know friends who have come to grief through unbridled cocaine consumption, but they also know people who have taken a bit here and a bit there and continued to finish their degrees and get good jobs in the City. It is significant that the common response to the news of cocaine finds at Westminster was amusement rather than scandal.

Heroin alone continues to cast an evil shadow. People who take cocaine and cannabis reassure themselves that they are not taking heroin. The influential classes still largely agree with the perception of MP Paul Flynn that if you take heroin, you will end up 'lying in a gutter with a needle sticking out of you'. In the mist of shifting attitudes to drug use, heroin shines out like a comforting lightship, a firm guide to perils that must be avoided. For over twenty years the Manchester agency Lifeline has been successfully counselling safe use among young drug users with a litany of dos and don'ts. Prominent among the don'ts have been two rules: (1) don't inject; (2) don't take heroin. Even such a streetwise agency as Lifeline has consistently seen heroin as the ultimate bad drug.

It is our contention that all this is beginning to change. Heroin is beginning to move upwards in society. For many years in the UK heroin use has grown at a rate of twenty per cent per year, in spite of all government policies. Very recent figures indicate that over the last two years this growth may be finally slowing down or even stopping.[16] This would be excellent news, if it were maintained. Nonetheless, we should be prepared for an equally likely scenario, that the growth in heroin use will pick up again and continue at the same rate as over the last two decades. Inevitably such a spread would begin to take in relatives and friends of policy makers if not the policy makers themselves. Inevitably also it would take in people who because of education and social circumstance are able to use heroin in a restrained and undestructive fashion. This would cause a gradual shift in the image of the drug. The idea that heroin is invariably evil would be replaced by the idea that it can sometimes lead to bad consequences, an idea which we have shown is very much nearer to the truth.

We also believe that this will happen at a speed, which will take most people by surprise. The laws of maths are such that a 20 per cent annual growth means a rapidly steepening curve of the actual number using heroin. This is geometric not arithmetic growth. It just takes twelve years at 20 per cent annual growth for the number to increase tenfold. Geometric growth can mimic a sudden eruption when it bursts through a threshold of social visibility. It suddenly starts being used by people in your street and being handed around at parties given by your friends or those of your children.

Moreover, it is the nature of British society that the influential fashion-leaders are closely connected to the ruling classes. Prince Charles' godson is in trouble for sniffing cocaine in fashionable night-clubs. Tony Blair's friend James Palumbo owns the Ministry of Sound, a popular night club and well-known venue for drug experimentation.[17] Heroin does not have to conquer the whole country before it can influence the policy-makers. There is a fifth column already established in the capital. We foresee heroin leapfrogging quickly from deprived neighbourhoods to London bars and night clubs, and becoming a drug of common use in influential circles well before it spreads to Middle England.

We believe that cannabis will prove to be a gateway drug, but not in the sense that those who take cannabis inevitably proceed to use cocaine and heroin. Acceptance of cannabis will act as a gateway to a general revision of thought about drug categories and to the eventual acceptance of cocaine and later of heroin. Cocaine will also prove a key factor in the spread of heroin. The drugs go well together. Heroin is excellent for smoothing out the crashdown after cocaine. Cocaine is excellent for getting one going after the relaxed torpor of heroin. Many heroin users started off with a cocaine habit. As cocaine spreads through the prosperous quarters of our cities, heroin will inevitably follow in its wake.

Heroin is also perhaps the drug of choice for coping with the insecurities of modern life. Jazz musicians have long appreciated its soothing properties:

> Heroin reduces the anxiety of social life, especially in an underground art and rock scene simultaneously characterised by chronic insecurity and outsize egos, relentless competition and the stark alternatives of sudden success and permanent obscurity.[18]

But these days everybody faces chronic insecurity, sudden success and permanent obscurity. The world of the London businessman increasingly resembles that of the New York musician.

Moreover, there is a drift away from political activity and growing helplessness in the face of global problems such as climate change, famine and terrible wars. Heroin is the ideal drug for opting out, if only on a temporary basis. Lou Reed's lyrics to 'Heroin' are also a hymn to political apathy.[19] Cometh the hour, cometh the drug. If heroin is readily available and fulfils a need, then without doubt it will be gratefully used.

All this may seem to conflict with what we wrote in Chapter 6 about the tightening of legal measures against drug misuse. But the band is at its tightest just before its snaps. These measures probably represent a last desperate attempt to halt an inevitable transformation. Their failure will ultimately hasten the move towards acceptance. It is not surprising that a Home Affairs Select Committee has now been established in the House of Commons to consider, among other issues, 'whether existing drug policies work, what would be the effect of decriminalisation ... and whether decriminalisation is desirable'.[20] We believe it likely that this committee and its successors will gradually move us down the route towards full legalisation.

Organised crime and state corruption

There is a much greater threat to the world than an increase in the number of people who use drugs. This is the large-scale organised crime that is intimately associated with their distribution. This problem is so huge that it threatens the integrity of whole countries. It is a threat as serious as famine and climate change. It can only be overcome if drug distribution is taken away from gangster organisations and handed over to legitimate authorities.

In 1997 drug turnover represented 8 per cent of international trade and at least \$120 billion were laundered through banks. This huge flow of money inevitably produces economic distortions which undermine sound finance. For example, investments in bogus companies undermine genuine business, so the governmental control of money supply is disrupted. By 2004 the world wide value of investments from the drug trade will be £1,000 billion, which is equal to the world's gold stocks. In other words the world's banks will be kept afloat on a raft of criminal proceeds.[21]

Corruption becomes endemic at the highest levels in government. Myanmar, Indonesia, Colombia and Afghanistan are just a few examples of countries whose rule is grossly distorted by the drug trade. The 1980 'cocaine coup' in Bolivia took place at the behest of drug traffickers.[22] The dangers were well expressed by Senator Gomez Hurtado, Colombian Ambassador to France:

> Forget about drug deaths and acquisitive crime, about addiction and AIDS; all this pales into insignificance before the prospect facing the liberal democracies of the West, like a rabbit in the headlights of an oncoming car. The income of the drug barons is an annual \$254 thousand million, greater than the American defence budget. With this financial power they can suborn all the institutions of the State, and if the State resists, with this fortune they can purchase the firepower to outgun it. We are threatened with a return to the Dark Ages of rule by the gang.[23]

It is tempting to see these problems as belonging to distant underdeveloped countries. But the UK has the largest consumer market for illicit drugs in Europe. The Office of National Statistics estimated that British users spend £7.5 billion on drugs a year and that the absence of this figure from official accounts produces 'a distorted picture of the British economy'.[24] Moreover, Britain has become the hub of the European drug trade and London the main centre for money laundering.[7]

British narco-traders are no longer the petty rulers of deprived neighbourhoods. The modern example is someone like Curtis Warren.[7] Known as a real-estate tycoon in Manchester and Liverpool, he moved to Holland to avoid the attention of the British police. Following his arrest in 1996, police recovered in Amsterdam seventy-five kilograms of heroin and five tons of marijuana, along with firearms and grenades. At his trial he revealed that he obtained cocaine directly from Colombia, heroin from Turkey, marijuana from Morocco and ecstasy from Holland. This is major international trading, but only made possible by widespread corruption of police and officials. Bribery or its analogues reach the highest levels. Drug-trade connections have often been alleged among the very rich men who have generously funded the Conservative Party.[25]

Moreover, drug dealers are the paymasters of the majority of the world's wars. Almost every secessionary movement is funded through drug sales, whether in Africa, South America or Asia. Again, this is not a distant problem that we can comfortably ignore. The Irish Republican Army (IRA) makes sure its backyard is clean of heroin by the kneecapping and punishment beating of rival dealers in Ulster. There is very little heroin use in Belfast. But the story is different in the Republic of Ireland. Dublin's heroin epidemic has much to do with the funds needed by the IRA to purchase its rocket launchers and Kalashnikovs.[26] The IRA also has close connections with other terrorist and criminal movements, from the Basque separatists to the Sicilian mafiosi. The arrest in August 2001 of IRA officers in Colombia has helped to reveal the organisation's connections with the Revolutionary Armed Forces of Colombia (FARC) and their terrorist war against the government, and also the IRA's involvement in Cuba's attempts to control lucrative drug routes to North America and Europe.[27] Trafficking in arms and trafficking in drugs are intimately connected.

What would happen if heroin were legal?

For all these reasons we believe that some kind of legalisation will arrive sooner rather than later. The 'war on drugs' is clearly not succeeding. Concerns about international corruption, war and financial stability will become more and more pressing. At the same time, social changes will make the use of heroin less frightening and more understandable. The balance will change and the scale will tip down suddenly on the side of acceptance.

We believe that changes are happening very quickly and that, as a result, there will be serious and influential pressure for the legalisation of heroin within the next ten years. In fact, we predict that some steps towards decriminalisation will have occurred within this space of time. It is for this reason that we have attempted to provide a dispassionate review of heroin, its history and its properties. A serious debate can only be based on accurate knowledge. It allows one to look ahead and visualise a society in which heroin use is legal and to speculate whether or not this would be disastrous.

It must be said first of all that legalisation does not mean the abandonment of all control. In fact some types of control are only possible when a drug is brought within the scope of the law. The quality of the drug can be controlled, and the manufacturing and marketing process can be regulated. A ban on supply to minors can be instituted much more effectively. Use in particular places can be barred, as happens at present with tobacco smoking in railway carriages and restaurants. On this analogy, it would probably be much easier to clamp down on the social nuisance of discarded needles and syringes if consumption of the drug itself were legal.

Economic measures can also be brought to bear. Of all government measures, the only one that has been shown consistently to reduce the use of a drug is to increase the level of taxation.[28] It is one of the best-established findings in alcohol research that the level of consumption of alcohol in Britain over 250 years has almost exactly mirrored the real cost of alcohol. Unfortunately there is a limit beyond which raising cost ceases to be useful, because contraband becomes irresistibly attractive. This level has probably been reached already in British tobacco taxation.[29] But, nonetheless, the ability to tax heroin would raise large amounts of revenue and would provide the government with one effective tool to moderate excessive use.

If production takes place once more in authorised factories, then in theory supply can be controlled. Under the Bratt system in Sweden all alcohol was sold through shops owned by government monopoly and customers were only allowed to purchase amounts considered to be reasonable. Their allocated ration was recorded in a 'motbok'. A panel could suspend the right to buy alcohol completely in cases of persistent inebriation. In theory, heroin could be sold in this manner. Unfortunately this system has now disappeared in Sweden, due largely to free-trade requirements of the European Union. It must be admitted that in the modern world there is a limit to which any country can control these issues independently.

Methods of controlling legal drugs have not always been applied energetically because of widespread social acceptance of their use. Tobacco is now more generally recognised as a dangerous drug and therefore governments feel empowered to exercise stronger control, while continuing to permit its use. Measures adopted include the banning of advertising, stricter prohibition of sales to minors and the compulsory printing of health messages and pictures on packets of cigarettes. Recently a UK parliamentary committee has recommended the establishment of a 'nicotine regulation authority'. It would bring the activities of cigarette manufacturers under statutory control, particularly in regard to marketing, advertising, sponsorship, packaging, labelling, heath claims, brand stretching, harm reduction, product development and the use of additives.[30] It is obvious from this lengthy list that there is much more that could be done to protect smokers from the harmful effects of their addiction.

But others have argued that the government should go further. Smokers are addicted to nicotine, but it is not the nicotine that causes most of the physical damage. Cigarettes kill because of the action of tar and the other combustion products of tobacco. There are 13 million smokers in Britain, most of whom will never overcome their addiction. Legislation should therefore encourage the development of alternative products which can deliver uncontaminated nicotine at a dose and rate comparable with cigarettes and in a way that is commercially and socially acceptable. These might be aerosols or perhaps smart skin patches from which the rate of nicotine release could be controlled by the wearer. According to a recent editorial in the *British Medical Journal*,

> The government has an immediate obligation to existing smokers in Britain, most of whom are amongst the most disadvantaged members of society ... . These people deserve protection against the activities of the tobacco industry and some safer solution to their nicotine addiction.[31]

Of course, exactly the same arguments could be applied to heroin addiction. Present policy is preventing addicts from getting hold of uncontaminated heroin and clean equipment, with severe consequences to their health. They are also drawn from 'the most disadvantaged members of society'. In fact, we think it is likely that the official attitudes to tobacco and heroin will gradually converge, the one becoming more tightly regulated and the other less so. Making nicotine illegal would never be feasible, but the lessons learnt in making its use safer will in time be applied to heroin.

The measures described above have either been shown to be effective to a certain degree or have some hope of carrying benefit in the future. They can only be applied if drug use is legal. While it remains illegal, governments have to rely instead on the police and the customs, neither of whom have had any clear success in reducing the spread of heroin use or increasing its cost. Legalising heroin would therefore increase control of heroin in some respects, such as quality and patterns of social use, without necessarily giving up controls that have proved effective.

Nonetheless, there is little doubt that there will be in future a large increase in the number of people using the drug, whether with or without legalisation. One calculation is that with legalisation it will increase eventually tenfold.[32] As we have said earlier, the recent rate of increase could lead to a tenfold expansion in twelve years without legalisation. In either case, use might then be similar to that of opium in the nineteenth century, except with far more control and regulation. At that time opium could be bought by anybody without prescription from chemists' shops. But, in spite of this uninhibited pattern of consumption, there was little social concern about opium misuse until late in the century, and then for complex reasons not necessarily related to public health.[33]

Would legal heroin be bad news for health?

It is uncertain what effect such an increase in heroin use would have on general health. Pharmaceutical heroin could be taken by snorting or by one of the more sophisticated methods described above. If injecting heroin, it should prove possible to avoid the terrible problems of infected and thrombosed veins which are so common today. Mostly these arise because people inject smoking heroin made partly soluble by cooking with acid. Pharmaceutical heroin hydrochloride dissolves instantly in small amounts of water. It can produce a hit if injected into the muscle rather than the vein. Patients prescribed this type of heroin are usually able to inject themselves for years without any venous damage or sepsis.

People already using heroin would be healthier than they are at present. Hopefully too there would be a move back to 'soothing cordials' and other oral preparations such as laudanum. But now there would be strict age regulations. Young children would not receive these drinks, in the same way they do not get given brandy today. The bottles would be clearly labelled with strength and content. Perhaps also there might be a return to opium smoking. It was after all suppression of this practice round the globe that led to heroin's dominance today. One old lady's reminiscences, taken from a US oral history project, tell us that this was not progress:

> There's nothing like a pipie [opium smoker]. They kept themselves immaculate – dresses, furs. I had a diamond, black mink coat, a Persian stole – whatever fur was, I had it because you wanted to look good. Nobody even knew I was a pipie. There was a million times difference between heroin and opium users, a million times. When I became a junkie, I lost my life.[34]

Health also suffers when self-care and presentation are neglected.

Death by overdose is a risk for heroin users, but an increase in heroin use would certainly not lead to a parallel increase in overdose. As we have argued in Chapter 7, overdose is largely a function of wildly irresponsible use of heroin in conjunction with other drugs by people with little commitment to normal life. The new heroin users would on the whole be people much better equipped to handle their habit responsibly.

Heroin-related health problems would probably increase, even if not to the same extent as consumption increased. But on the other hand there may be compensatory gains. For a start, one would hope that there would be less people in prison. Imprisonment has a substantial impact on the health of both convicts and their families. By making subsequent employment less likely, it continues to have a harmful effect after the sentence is finished. Prison is also a major reservoir of infection. More people developed HIV infection in one Scottish prison over a year than in the whole of Manchester and Liverpool.[35]

As more people use heroin there would be more discussion about safe ways to use the drug. The dangers of injecting would be discussed on Woman's Hour, in teenage magazines, in schools and in popular soaps. Everybody would know about hepatitis and AIDS, and the risks of using dirty equipment. Healthy models of safe use would develop. It is possible that public acceptance would actually reduce the spread of hepatitis. We have argued that heroin itself is a remarkably safe drug. The main danger comes from unhygienic injecting practice. Legalisation might reduce this risk.

Heroin use would also not necessarily be a straight addition to other drug use. It would have to find its niche in a crowded market-place. One drug that it might start displacing is alcohol. Both are sedative and relaxing. Although there are people who misuse both drugs, a lot of heroin users do not touch alcohol at all, even though they may originate from families with a long tradition of heavy drinking. Excessive alcohol is far more harmful to the system than heroin and productive of far more social disturbance. A moderate shift from alcohol to heroin could actually cause net gains in public health.

It is of some comfort that illicit drugs make only a small contribution to the overall burden of disease. A recent report attempted to quantify the global health burden posed by various risk factors in terms of 'disability adjusted life years' (DALYs), a measure that combined time lost due to both death and premature disability. Of DALYs, 16 per cent were caused by malnutrition, 7 per cent by poor sanitation and between 2 and 4 per cent each by unsafe sex, alcohol, air pollution, tobacco and occupational risk. All illicit drugs together accounted for less than 0.5 per cent.[36] Even if the health burden posed by illicit drugs increases, they will have a long way to go before they compete seriously with these other major killers. If the money now spent on the war against drugs was diverted to providing poor nations with improved sanitation and water supplies, then there might be some real hope of improved health across the world.

New medical treatments

Medical treatment should also improve as consumers became more articulate and demanding. Moreover, there would be ample money to fund research and treatment if taxation was raised on heroin use. Heroin treatment at present is not a priority for the pharmaceutical industry, but legalisation would bring it to the forefront of their business plans. There are already a number of new treatments in the pipeline. Their development would be accelerated.

The most promising avenue is what is called 'peripheral blockade'. A medicine is taken which blocks the effect of heroin and renders it useless. Naltrexone is a molecule very similar to heroin. It fits so neatly into opiate receptors that it occupies them in preference to heroin. But, while heroin stimulates the receptor when it clicks into place, naltrexone produces no reaction. If you take naltrexone after heroin, it will displace all the heroin molecules and send you into withdrawal. If you take it every day, your receptors will all be occupied and any heroin you take will have no effect. Naltrexone is an effective medicine for heroin addicts if it is taken every day. But in that 'if' lies a big problem. In spite of thirty years of trying, naltrexone has not proved successful in routine use because patients somehow forget to take it. Its best results have come from Singapore, where the tablet is administered daily by police staff. It seems to require this level of enforcement to make a difference. What may change this equation is the development of a naltrexone implant. This is surgically implanted in the abdominal wall every three months and is completely effective over that time in suppressing the heroin response. A couple of implants will take one through the period where one is most in danger of relapsing after detoxification. Official trials have not yet been carried out, but early results from pioneers are promising.

An alternative method of blockade is to use a vaccine. This uses the body's immune system to neutralise circulating heroin before it hits the brain. Scientists were developing such a vaccine twenty years ago, but work stopped after the discovery of naltrexone because it was thought the vaccine would become redundant. Now interest is reviving because of the successful development of a vaccine against cocaine. This uses 'passive' antibodies to break down circulating cocaine molecules. In other words, the antibodies are not those that the body makes itself but are prepared externally and injected. The result is that the immunity lasts about three months before the antibodies disappear. As with naltrexone, this is a very useful length of time to help someone recover from an oppressive habit. It is likely that work will start again soon on a heroin vaccine.[37]

The chemistry of craving is also beginning to be unravelled. The experience of craving is what leads addicts to relapse when they are trying to stay clean. Everyday experiences associated with drug use trigger these cravings, for example seeing spoons or needles, hearing conversation about drugs or being in the vicinity where one usually scores. But it has also become clear that this experience of craving is connected to changes in brain chemistry that occur with prolonged use of a drug. Correcting these changes may reduce craving and thus prevent relapse. So far no one has developed a drug which reduces craving for heroin, but acamprosate and bupropion have recently been introduced into the market and are prescribed to reduce craving for alcohol and nicotine. Apart from helping addicts, they have also signalled to the pharmaceutical industry that investing in addiction treatment could be very profitable. It will not be long before a medicine appears that can reduce the craving for heroin.

Ibogaine

No survey of future treatments can ignore the African dream-root *tabernathe iboga*.[38] This has been used in the Gabon since time immemorial as an initiation rite into the Bwiti cult. After months of careful preparation, the acolytes drink a preparation of iboga root. They then vomit and gradually sink into a trance. Music, dancing and colourful shapes increase the effect. Spiritual 'parents' guide them through a series of hallucinations which gradually reveal to them the hidden wisdom of the cult. Breathing slows and a deep sleep ensues. On recovery, they feel fresh and relaxed, but also as if something has changed totally inside.

This root was bought back to France at the beginning of the century. The active ingredient was crystallised in 1901 and called ibogaine. In low doses it was found to be a mild stimulant. Before the war, doctors used it to treat their 'tired all the time' patients. Like all the best drugs it also got involved in a doping scandal when cyclists started using it in the Tour de France cycle race.

American psychotherapists became interested in the 1960s. At this time they were exploring the use of LSD as a way of unlocking hidden memories and resolving unacknowledged psychic conflicts. A psychotherapist named Claude Naranjo started prescribing ibogaine and reported that it produced not so much hallucinations as an 'oneirophrenic' dream-like state in which the subject could be guided towards visualising in a state of calmness scenes which would otherwise have been deeply upsetting. Naranjo thought therefore that it was ideally suited for psychotherapy and would help patients come to terms with unbearable trauma from the past.[39] Unfortunately this type of research disappeared when LSD became a banned drug.

In 1968 an American named Howard Lotsof heard about this drug and thought that it might help him overcome his heroin addiction. He managed to get supplies from the Gabon. To his surprise he found that, after taking it on one occasion, not only did he stop using heroin but that he also experienced no withdrawals or cravings. He claims not to have used heroin since and considers himself cured. Since that time he has been conducting an evangelical and entrepreneurial campaign to get ibogaine adopted into conventional medicine.

A fascinating conference on ibogaine was held in New York in the autumn of 1999.[40] There were presentations from scientists who showed that ibogaine reduced withdrawal symptoms in animals and also appeared to reverse signs suggestive of heroin addiction, such as an established preference for a cage in which heroin had been supplied. For pharmacists the race was on to produce a related substance that would have the same positive effect without the nausea and hallucinations. The pharmaceutical industry was not going to market a drug which caused an 'oneirophrenic state', however attractive to psychotherapists. On the other hand, there were groups of therapists and reformed addicts who argued that the vomiting and the hallucinatory experiences were an essential part of the cure. These groups had attempted to reproduce some of the ritual aspects of Bwiti, albeit modified for a secular society. These people saw unrestrained heroin use as a kind of existential solution for deep personal and social problems. A personal transformation was necessary to move away from heroin use and this required a quasi-religious ritual with support from those who had already made the journey.

This belief is supported by research which shows that people kick their addiction when they are ready to do so. Neither criminal sanctions nor technological fixes are sufficient by themselves to produce a cure, but both can be effective if applied at the right time. Hopefully more widespread use of heroin would lead to wiser treatment of those who had lost control. Cure cannot be imposed or produced by a tablet. Indeed unbridled use of drugs is not really a medical problem at all. It is a life choice, which can only be challenged by the realistic offer of better alternatives, backed up with a viable route for their achievement. The role of medicine is to provide a bridge to the other side, but drug users must want to cross over and must find it worthwhile when they arrive.

Conclusion – and a nice cup of tea

We predict that heroin use will continue to spread and that, before very many years have passed, it will achieve acceptance and some degree of decriminalisation. As a therapeutic exercise we have attempted to face up to this frightening prospect in much the same way as Dr Strangelove in the Peter Sellers film learnt to stop worrying and to love the Bomb. We have found the prospect not as terrifying as it first appears. Health problems will probably increase, but not as much as many people fear. On the other hand, taking the drug trade away from gangsters will have a hugely positive effect on public finances and public order.

It is fitting that an English book about drugs should end with a digression on the subject of tea. Oasis singer Noel Gallagher notoriously remarked on a radio show that taking drugs was 'like getting up and having a cup of tea in the morning'. He also added, with some prescience, that 'there's people in the House of Parliament, man, who are bigger heroin and cocaine addicts than anyone in this room right now'.[41] He probably did not realise that, once upon a time, tea also had to fight for acceptance and there were many who attacked it as a danger to public health:

> What an army has gin and tea destroyed! How often have the spirits of both parents and children been forced to quit their bodies, when these are set in a blaze with gin; or the springs of life lose their powers by the enervating powers of tea![42]

Even so sensible a commentator as William Cobbett had serious concerns about the dangers of tea:

> Tea-drinking is a troublesome and pernicious habit. I view tea-drinking as a destroyer of health, an enfeebler of the frame, an engenderer of effeminacy and laziness, a debaucher of the youth, and a maker of misery in old age.[43]

Like heroin, tea arrived in Europe as a medicine.[44] It was originally appreciated by the rich as something exotic, but soon caused concern when it spread to the lower classes. In time, however, governments realised it was a valuable source of trade and taxation. Indeed, it was the need to pay for Chinese tea that inspired British merchants with the happy idea of importing opium to China.[45] Later on, the tea plantations in India contributed greatly to the wealth of the British Empire.

It may seem absurd to compare heroin and tea (though tea is a common slang-term for marijuana). But tea contains many strong stimulants. The reason it appears harmless is because we have learnt to use it in a safe manner, drinking it in a weak infusion. Not many tea users have the pioneering spirit of one of our patients, who claimed to generate reliable hallucinations by smoking teabags. But consider what happened when tea first arrived in Tunisia in the 1930s, brought in by itinerant workers to a naïve population. A Tunisian physician was shocked by what he saw:

> Throughout the Kingdom, from North to South, from East to West, we now find groups of our compatriots, seated round low round tables specially made for the purpose, drinking tea almost continuously. The quantity of tea used is so great that it produces a liquid black as tar, and of a syrupy consistency. Delicate throats could not tolerate even a couple of mouthfuls! ... At present in Tunisia, tea is the main, if not the only stimulus for late-night parties. In town, these gatherings take place in seedy Moorish cafes. Nonetheless, the dangers from lack of hygiene in these clubs are less than those found in the villages. There the villagers spend long hours in disgusting hovels, breathing polluted air. They are at the mercy of tuberculosis.
>
> The abuse of tea has taken on the characteristics of a plague – it is not only confined to men, but has even spread to women and children. The situation is becoming very dangerous. From the medical point of view, observations collected from many natives throughout the kingdom indicate the existence of severe maladies of the nervous and circulatory systems.
>
> I have previously noted that tea abuse among our Moslem compatriots takes the form of an extreme passion, inflamed by an imperious and irresistible craving. When the tea-hour approaches and they feel the need to drink, the natives appear completely incapable.

They must at all costs drink their ration of tea to regain their normal calm. They will even cut back on their intake of food rather than sacrifice their tea! It is very likely this malnutrition which causes the sickly complexion of our country folk, who before looked so healthy!

The thefts they now commit are motivated by the need to satisfy their passion for tea. ... One evening during a severe winter this native sold his only good warm blanket to satisfy his craving for tea. This blanket was the only protection from the cold for himself, his wife and his poor little children who were for the most part sickly and suffered from rickets ... [46]

While doctors were worrying about tea, the attitude to cannabis in Tunisia was more relaxed:

The sale of chopped hemp ready for smoking (*takrouri*) is a state monopoly like the sale of tobacco, salt, gunpowder and matches. The *Direction des monopoles* every year fixes the area of authorized plantations and issues cultivation permits. It buys the complete crop of whole plants from the producers. The Tunis Tobacco Factory prepares *takrouri*, by cleaning, chopping and sifting. It divides it up into packets of five grammes which are sold, without any formalities, in all the tobacco shops of the Tunis Regency. In 1937, 6,387 kilogrammes of *takrouri* were sold, i.e. 1,277,400 packets, at 2 frs 35 centimes each.[47]

No doubt many young Tunisians argued at the time that drinking a cup of tea was no worse than getting up in the morning and smoking a pipe of *takrouri*. And their elders would have responded with anger and ridicule. Such is the topsy-turvy world of *your drug/my drug*.

The histories of tobacco, cocoa and coffee are surprisingly similar to tea. They started off as medicines and delicacies for the rich. They then spread to the lower orders. This generated huge concern and a vain attempt at repression. With the passage of years the state became more relaxed about their dangers and more appreciative of their potential role in trade and the generation of taxes. People learnt to use them more wisely. The drugs then became an integral part of the social fabric; their benefits were enjoyed and the harms they caused were tolerated and almost ignored.[48] There is no doubt that in time heroin will travel the same route to public acceptance. We believe this will happen sooner rather than later, and that on balance it will be beneficial.

Notes

1 Wilkinson, Francis (1999) 'Time to wipe the drug barons' smile', *The Times* (8 November), p. 17.
2 Bennett, William J. (1990) 'Should drugs be legalised?', *Readers Digest* (March): 22–40.
3 Powderject homepage at www.powderject.com.
4 Dobson, R. (1998) 'Smart needles home in on veins to make injections painless', *Sunday Times (Innovation supplement)* (6 December), p. 14.
5 For more information about these developments, see *Medicines by Design: the Biological Revolution in Pharmacology* at the National Institute of General Medical Science website www.nigms.nih.gov/news/science_ed/medbydes.html.
6 Egginton, R. and Parker, H. (2000) *Hidden Heroin Users*, Manchester: Manchester University Press. p. 8.
7 Observatoire Geopolitique des Drogues (1999) *Annual Report 1997–1998*, Paris: OGD, p. 26.
8 Wintour, P. (2000) 'Widdecombe forced to backtrack on cannabis', *The Guardian* (9 October), pp. 1–2.
9 'An Experiment With Cannabis', *The Daily Telegraph* (30 March 2000), p. 31.
10 Thorp, R. (1956) *Viper. The Confessions of a Drug-Addict*, London: Robert Hale.
11 Chittenden, M. (2000) 'Cocaine user snorted drug in Lords loo', *The Sunday Times* (5 November): 2G.
12 'Analysis and Report of Original Documentary Evidence Concerning the Use of Opium in India,' *The British Medical Journal* (1893): 1175-6.
13 King James I (1604) *Counterblaste to Tobacco*, London: Robert Barker.
14 Peele, S. (1998) 'The results for drug reform goals of shifting from interdiction/punishment to treatment', *International Journal of Drug Policy* 9: 43–56.
15 Graham, H. Der G. (1999) 'Patterns and predictors of smoking cessation among British women', *Health Promotion International* 14: 231–9.
16 To judge from previous temporary pauses in growth a permanent slowdown is unlikely. Predicting the future is impossible, but we suspect that developments described in this chapter are not likely to be put back by no more than ten years at most as a result of this apparent slowdown. See: United Nations Office for Drug Control and Crime Prevention (2001) *Global Illicit Drug Trends,* New York: UNODCCP
17 Although he claims his organisation vigorously opposes the use of drugs, this is hardly consistent with the contents of the house magazine *Ministry*. In August 1998 readers were invited to identify a real ecstasy tablet among a large number of other pills on a colour double-page. An article also deplored the poor quality of the latest batch of 'dove' ecstasy pills. In May 1999 it ran a six-page special on how to grow cannabis. In March 2000 clubbers could enjoy a ten-page drug special including lots of fun reports from people describing their 'most memorable drug experiences'.
18 A.M. (1994) 'Listening to heroin', *Village Voice*: 25–30.
19 See Victor Bockris (1995) *Lou Reed: the Biography*, London: Vintage Books.

20 Home Affairs Select Committee (2001) *The Government's drug policy? Is it working?*, London: Houses of Parliament Press Notice (24 July).

21 Lashmar, P. (1998) 'Shooting up', *Independent: Review* (16 July): 1.

22 Corn, David (1991) 'The CIA and the Cocaine Coup', *The Nation* (7 October): 404–6.

23 Hurtado, G. (1993) Speech at American Drug Policy Foundation Conference, Baltimore. Quoted in J. Marks (1994) 'Drug legalisation: Letter from (South) America', *The Lancet* 343: 296–7. See also G. Hurtado (1993) *La Tragedia de la Droga (The tragedy of drugs)*, Bogota: University of Sergio Arboleda.

24 Office of National Statistics (1998) 'Developing a methodology for measuring illegal activity in the UK national accounts', *Economic Trends* (July).

25 For example, it is claimed that a £1 million donation was made to the party in June 1994 by Chinese millionaire Ma Sik-Chun, who had fled from Taiwan after being charged with drug trafficking. See 'The ultimate betrayal? Tories took money from a heroin baron', *The Independent* (20 January 1998): 1. This accusation was also made in Parliament by MP Dennis Skinner. See House of Commons Hansard Debates (13 November 1997): part 6. It has also been claimed that much of ex-party chairman Lord Ashcroft's fortune comes from the operations of banks in Belize which are havens for money laundering by drug traffickers. He used this money to make large donations to the party. See 'US raises crime fears in Ashcroft tax haven', *Guardian* (4 June 2001).

26 See, for example, 'IRA may allow drugs if it is given a cut of profits', *Irish Times* (11 March 1998), p. 1.

27 McGrory, D. and Arostegui, M. (2001) 'IRA men were teaching high-tech bomb skills', *The Times* (18 August): 2.

28 Institute of Alcohol Studies (1999) *Alcohol:Tax and Price and Public Health*, London: Institute of Alcohol Studies.

29 It is calculated that in 1999 a quarter to a third of all cigarettes smoked in England had been illegally imported, at a cost of £2.5 billion to the revenue. See A. Rowell and C. Bates (2000) *Tobacco smuggling in the UK*, London: Action on Smoking and Health. Moreover, most inhabitants of deprived areas view tobacco smuggling as 'a legitimate way to challenge the perceived injustice of regressive tobacco taxation'. See S. Wiltshire, A. Bancroft, A. Amos and O. Parry (2001) ' "They're doing people a service" – qualitative study of smoking, smuggling and social deprivation', *British Medical Journal* 323: 203–7.

30 House of Commons Health Committee (2000) *The Tobacco Industry and the Health Risks of Smoking*, London: Stationery Office.

31 Britton, J. and McNeill, A. (2001) 'Why Britain needs a nicotine regulation authority', *British Medical Journal* 322: 1,077–8.

32 Working Party of the Royal College of Psychiatrists and the Royal College of Physicians (2000) *Drugs, Dilemmas and Choices*, London: Gaskell, 23rd August, p. 255.

33 Berridge, V. and Edwards, G. (1987) *Opium and the People: opiate use in nineteenth century England*, New Haven: Yale University Press.

34 Courtwright, D., Joseph, H. and Des Jarlais, D. (1989) *Addicts who survived*, Knoxville: University of Tennessee Press.

35 Taylor, A. *et al.* (1995) 'Outbreak of HIV infection in a Scottish prison', *British Medical Journal* 310: 289–92.

36 *The 10/90 Report on Health Research 2000*, Geneva: Global Forum on Health Research. Available at www.globalforumhealth.org.

37 National Institute on Drug Abuse (1998) *A Summary of Peripheral Blockers as Treatments for Substance Abuse and Dependence*, Rockville: National Institute on Drug Abuse.

38 For a huge amount of literature and information about ibogaine, see www.ibogaine.org.

39 Naranjo, C. (1973) *The healing journey. New approaches to consciousness*, New York: Pantheon.

40 New York University Conference on Ibogaine, 5–6 November 1999.

41 Wallace, R. & Dodd, S., 'E's got a point', *The Mirror*, 31 January 1997, p. 5.

42 Hanway, Jonas (1756) 'An essay on tea, considered as pernicious to health, obstructing industry and impoverishing the nation', in *A Journal of Eight Days' Journey from Portsmouth to Kingston upon Thames*, London: H. Woodfall (1757), p. 89. The book was later reviewed somewhat sceptically by Samuel Johnson, although he started his article by confessing his own tea addiction:

> He (Mr Hanway) is to expect little justice from the author of this extract, a hardened and shameless tea-drinker, who has, for twenty years, diluted his meals with only the infusion of this fascinating plant; whose kettle has scarcely time to cool; who with tea amuses the evening, with tea solaces the midnight, and, with tea, welcomes the morning.

See Samuel Johnson (1757) 'A Review of a *Journal of Eight Days' Journey*', *The Literary Magazine* 2: 13.

43 Cobbett, William (1823) *Cottage Economy*, London: J.M. Cobbett, Section 29. The contrary view is that the tannin in tea was a crucial antiseptic that prevented dysentery in crowded urban environments and thereby enabled the industrial revolution to take place in England. See A. Ahuja (2000) 'Did tea and beer make Britain great?', *The Times* (10 May): 12–13.

44 In the early days a distinguished Dutch doctor advised drinking a minimum of eight cups a day and claimed that fifty cups a day was even better for your health. It will come as no surprise to hear that he was receiving a backhander from the importers. See Rudi Matthee (1995) 'Exotic Substances', in R. Porter and M. Teich (eds) *Drugs and Narcotics in History*, Cambridge: Cambridge University Press.

45 Levinthal, C.F. (1985) 'Milk of paradise/milk of hell – the history of ideas about opium', *Perspectives in Biology and Medicine* 28: 561–77.

46 Dinguizli, M.B. (1927) 'Un nouveau fleau social: le théisme en Tunisie' ('A new social plague: tea addiction in Tunisia'), *Bulletin Academique de Medicine* 97: 423–9 (our translation from the French). Russell Pasha was later worried about an outbreak of tea addiction in Egypt. He feared that it might replace heroin addiction, which he had managed to suppress (see Chapter 4 of this book; E.W. Adams (1937) *Drug Addiction*, Oxford: Oxford University Press, p. 34).

47 Bouquet, J. (1951) 'Cannabis', *Bulletin of Narcotics* 4: 22–45.

48 See Matthee (1995).

Index

References to notes are followed by n